EBOLA CRISIS
Panic or Pandemic?

What You Need To Know For Survival

Georgia Begnaud

Disclaimer

Although the author has made every effort to ensure that the information in this book is accurate and current- relief efforts in the field are happening in real-time and our knowledge about Ebola disease is changing rapidly. The author disclaims any liability for loss, injury, damage, or disruptions caused by errors or omissions which may result from negligence, accident, or incorrect information on websites. The author recommends the CDC website as the definitive source for ongoing information about the Ebola pandemic in Western Africa. The author is not a physician and the information in this book is not to be used as a substitute for medical evaluation, diagnosis, or treatment. Please consult your physician, pharmacist, or health care provider if you have concerns or questions that require medical advice.

Table of Contents

Introduction

Ebola is a virulent disease with a mortality rate of 60-90% in people who are infected. The people who are at the greatest risk of exposure and disease are family members and health care workers who are caring for patients with active Ebola disease.

Ebola disease was first diagnosed in Zaire and the Congo in 1976. There have been 25 reported outbreaks of Ebola disease since 1976 with approximately 1850 cases and 1200 deaths. That gives a historical mortality rate from Ebola disease of 64.8%. Most of the outbreaks in the past were rapidly contained and the number of cases were low. Transmission of Ebola disease did not progress beyond the region that was affected.

The current Ebola epidemic is unlike any outbreak in the past. There have been five times more cases in 2014 than the total number of cases in history. Ebola disease is infecting large numbers of people in three African nations- Guinea, Liberia, and Sierra Leone. Case numbers are rising rapidly in Mali. There are isolated cases in other African nations. There have been 5 confirmed cases in the United States- 4 were health care workers caring for Ebola infected patients. Two of these patients died which gives a 40% mortality rate in the United States.

Many people are anxious about being exposed and becoming infected. There is a lot of information that is causing fear and panic. Is it justified? Are we on the verge of a global pandemic? Should we all wear masks and stay home? What is a reasonable response to the information you hear? What is your risk of disease? What do you need to know?

This book is a summary of what we know about Ebola disease today. We are learning more every day. The primary goal is to prevent a worldwide Ebola pandemic. Herculean efforts are underway to discover an effective vaccine and to find better ways of treating patients who have Ebola disease.

My goal is to help you understand Ebola disease and your risk of infection. Information is power and it gives perspective. I will review and dissect the Ebola literature and organize the information in a way that allows you to find the information you want rapidly. I will not use long words and medical mumbo-jumbo that is irrelevant and unclear. Each chapter contains important information. The conclusion will summarize the Ebola crisis and suggest a reasonable plan of action to take.

Thank you for reading this book. I hope you enjoy it and find it helpful. If the book has helped to answer your questions and clarify your response to Ebola- please leave a review on Amazon to help others who are also trying to find information and answers.

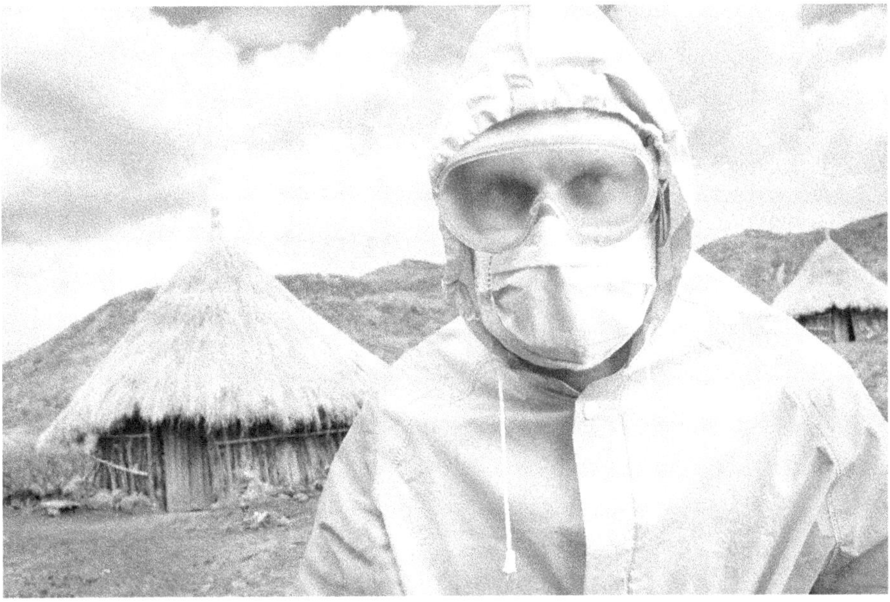

Part 1
Ebola Disaster

Chapter 1
How Serious is Ebola Disease?

Many of the statistics that I use come from the CDC website at http://www.cdc.gov/vhf/ebola and the World Health Organization (WHO) website at http://www.who.int/csr/disease/ebola.

The current statistics from the CDC updated on December 9, 2014 show:

- Total cases- 17,800
- Lab confirmed cases- 11,182
- Total deaths- 6,331
- Mortality- 57 % of confirmed cases

Mortality rates allow us to measure the **virulence** of a disease. Ebola disease overwhelms the immune system of the host and is lethal in about 60% of patients. Ebola is an extremely virulent disease with a high mortality rate.

Another important metric to study is the **spread rate**. This is a measure of how rapidly a disease is spreading. The spread rate is reported as an R value. It measures the disease's ability to spread to others who are not infected. An R of 1 means that each infected person will transmit the virus to one other person during the course of his infection.

- R=1- means a disease will continue to grow at the current rate.
- R > 1- the disease is still growing. The higher the R value the more rapidly the disease is spreading.
- R < 1- the disease is being controlled. Its growth is slowing and the epidemic is being contained. The R value should steadily decrease as the people with the disease recover or die.

- R=0- there are no more cases being discovered and the disease has run its course.

In the West African Ebola outbreak of 2014- the R has been as high as 2- it is currently reported as 1.8. That is an exponential growth rate. Let's put it into perspective. One of the most devastating infections in the past was the Spanish flu in 1918. One hundred million people died and disease was widespread across the globe. The R was 2.

An Ebola infection usually lasts about a month. An R value of 1.8 means that Ebola cases could double every 20- 25 days. CDC and WHO statistics indicate that Ebola disease rates are under-reported by a factor of 2.5. That means that for every case that is reported there are another 1.5 cases that are not reported. This shows that the scope of the Ebola crisis is much worse than the numbers indicate. The CDC website has projected from the current statistics that the number of cases in West Africa may reach as high as 550,000 by January 20, 2015 and that the actual numbers would probably exceed 1.4 million if disease reporting was more accurate.

Chapter 2
What is the difference between an outbreak, an epidemic, and a pandemic?

The term **outbreak** describes the sudden rise in the incidence of a disease, especially a harmful one. An **outbreak** is characterized by a disease's bypassing of measures to control it. Often, the difference between these terms is determined by the percentage of deaths caused by the disease

An **epidemic** is a disease that affects many people at the same time, such as the flu. The US Centers for Disease Control and Prevention's official definition of **epidemic** is: 'The occurrence of more cases of disease than expected in a given area or among a specific group of people over a particular period of time'.

A **pandemic** is a very extensive **epidemic**, like a plague, that is prevalent in a country, continent, or the world. There is also the word endemic, which is a disease native to a people or region, which is regularly or constantly found among a people or specific region.

These are the CDC guidelines for disease prevalence and classification. How would we classify the 2014 Ebola disease rates according to these definitions?

We have an Ebola outbreak that meets the CDC definition for an epidemic. It can also be defined as being pandemic in Western Africa. What is the risk for Ebola to spread to all nations of the world?

Definitive answers are hard to come by. You will hear many different conclusions but no one knows with absolute certainty what impact Ebola will have globally or how widespread and far-reaching it will extend.

Ebola is an international public health crisis now. Ebola virus is considered a level 4 bio-hazardous pathogen by the CDC and WHO.

Although Ebola disease is only pandemic in Western Africa now- the risk extends to all continents and countries of the world. Each nation must be proactive in guarding their borders. They must be prepared to manage Ebola infected patients safely and protect their citizens from infection. Their goals must be preventing Ebola virus transmission, isolating people with Ebola disease, and quarantine of all known contacts of patients with symptomatic Ebola disease.

Chapter 3
Hopelessness in Western Africa

(Quote) U. S. Ambassador to the United Nations, Samantha Power: "Ebola has no greater friend than fear. The virus thrives on it. We see fear in the affected countries... It is fear that leads community members to stigmatize survivors of the virus, or the relatives of those who have died, or even the health professionals and other people aiding in the response... A 24-year-old survivor in Guinea told me she had lived three lives: her life before Ebola; her life in the hell of her infection; and her life since recovering. She said the stigma she has suffered since beating Ebola has made her current life the hardest. The stigma had so affected her that she said she was amazed by President Obama's embrace of Nina Pham, the Texas nurse who was just cured of Ebola. When I went to give this young woman survivor a hug goodbye, though, she demurred and offered a fist bump. She did not seem yet to fully trust that she was cured or to recognize that she had done nothing wrong - only the virus had... It is fear that has caused some of those who develop a fever or other symptoms not to come forward to seek help, putting themselves and the people around them at greater risk. Fear that going to seek care will make them sicker, or that seeking help will alienate them from their communities... We also see fear in countries like my own (USA), whose active participation is critically important to bringing this outbreak under control. All over the world, governments and our fellow citizens are afraid that if we send doctors or nurses or soldiers or engineers or other volunteers to the affected countries, we will put our own communities at risk... The fear is understandable. Many of our countries, like those most affected, are dealing with Ebola for the first time, and it is a dangerous and terrifying virus... We must ask ourselves: twenty years from now, when we look back on this historic crossroads, will we want to say we left this fight to the people of the affected countries? Will we want to say we did not act because we thought others would win the fight without our help? Will we want to admit that fear held us back? If we will not want to give these answers when we are asked in twenty years - and make no mistake, we will all be asked - we have to do more."

Western Africa stands on the edge of the abyss. Here are a series of phrases that give us word pictures of the emotions felt in Western Africa. They help us feel the magnitude of the crisis at ground zero.

FEAR

Real
Overwhelming
Everyday

Don't talk to anyone
Don't trust anyone
Don't touch anyone

Stay far away
Pray

Wear a mask
Look around you
Stay out of crowds
Get off the streets
Hurry

Hospitals:

Overcrowded
Overworked
Overwhelmed
Exhausted
Fearful

Frustrated
No workers
No PPE
No resources
No supplies
Never ending stream of sick and dying patients
Hopeless

Ebola patients:

Victims
Dehumanized
Depersonalized
Demoralized
Stigmatized
Vulnerable
Helpless
Hopeless
Death waiting to happen

Western Africa:

Poverty
Isolation
Oppression
Civil war
Shunned
Stigmatized
Decimated by Ebola
Needs global aid NOW

Chapter 4
The Magnitude of Ebola in Western Africa

Ebola is currently the most feared disease in the world. The enemy is a virus that looks insignificant under a microscope. It is a living organism that looks like a coiled rope when it is magnified. Ebola virus is able to hide in reservoirs that we cannot identify. It multiplies, evolves, changes, mutates, and grows rapidly. The virus overwhelms the immune system of the infected person. It destroys the immune system...then it kills the person.

Ebola presents as an insignificant viral illness that mimics influenza but it rapidly progresses to a devastating illness that kills 60-90% of infected people. The traditional medical system of the civilized world has no answers- there are no anti-viral drugs that are effective, no treatment regimen that is proven to work, and no preventive vaccine.

Previous outbreaks of Ebola disease have almost exclusively affected Africa. The countries with the highest incidence of Ebola disease in the 2014 pandemic are Guinea, Libya, Sierra Leone, and Mali. They are among the poorest countries in the world. The daily wage for a worker is about $1.25. Their economies are supported by tourism, farming, hunting, and mining. All have been decimated by the 2014 Ebola pandemic.

The majority of the population lives in villages that are isolated and self-contained. There is no electricity. Clean water is a luxury. The climate is always hot and humid. Sanitation is poor and maintaining adequate hygiene is almost impossible. There are no septic systems and sewage lies in fields around the community. Large families live in primitive conditions and over-crowding is common. When someone in the family gets sick- everyone is at risk.

The African nations that are most affected by Ebola disease have been involved in civil wars for many years. They have lived with hatred and persecution and are frightened of strangers. They are anxious and fearful of anything they don't understand. Many are ignorant about Ebola virus including how it spreads and what to do to protect themselves and their family.

When someone becomes ill- they are cared for by their family and generally remain in their village. Medical infrastructure is limited- there are few physicians or hospitals and none are in the remote villages. Shamans and other natural healers of the tribes care for people who are ill according to tribal customs and rituals. People who die are buried using culturally acceptable burial ceremonies. Touching, hugging, wailing, kissing, and lying prostate on the body of the dead person are normal ways to grieve in their culture. These are meaningful parts of their mourning process. These rituals show love, respect, and honor to the person who died. Unfortunately- these practices also transmit Ebola virus and cause Ebola disease in healthy family members and villagers.

The WHO discourages taking care of Ebola patients in the home. It strongly recommends hospital care by a qualified team of medical professionals and health care workers using personal protective equipment and strict infection control measures. WHO guidelines require isolation of the infected patient, tracing of his contacts, and quarantine of anyone who was directly exposed to him. The goal is to keep Ebola virus from being transmitted to others who are not infected.

Villagers are suspicious of the motives of the people who are there to help. They believe that hate and genocide are behind their offers. They think that the government is persecuting them and the hospitals are experimenting on them.

African villagers feel frightened and anxious. They don't trust "outsiders" and are refusing to co-operate. They run away from medical authorities and law enforcement officers. They hide their sick family members so they won't be taken to hospitals. They are afraid that their loved ones will die among strangers and be buried in ways that are not acceptable to them. They believe that sending anyone from their family to the hospital is a death sentence for their loved one and that he will never be seen alive again.

These are some of the reasons why Ebola disease has become pandemic in Western Africa and why it continues to spread like wildfire through the villages and the bush. Poverty, fear, ignorance, isolation, distrust, lack of medical infrastructure and resources- all of these factors are contributing to the rapid spread of Ebola disease.

Capital cities and congested urban areas in Guinea, Liberia, Sierra Leone, and Mali have been infected with Ebola disease during the 2014 Ebola pandemic. Hospitals are full to capacity. There are inadequate numbers of hospitals and health care workers. There are critical shortages of medical supplies and personal protective equipment. None of these countries have the ability to manage a pandemic of this size and complexity.

584 health care workers have been infected and 329 have died from Ebola disease. That gives a mortality rate of 57% among health care workers who were infected while providing health care to patients with Ebola disease. Despite using PPE and stringent infectious control measures- health care workers are still being infected and dying of Ebola disease.

We live in a mobile society and have the ability to travel anywhere in the world. People who are exposed to the disease are buying airline tickets and traveling to countries with better health care systems. People who are in Western Africa on business are returning home. There is great risk that people who are leaving Western Africa may have been exposed to Ebola virus. They may be in the incubation period and not showing symptoms of disease. These people could reach their destinations before becoming sick. Early disease symptoms mimic influenza but patients are contagious and shedding Ebola virus as soon as any symptoms occur. They can expose and infect people as they conduct their usual routines of work, church, and social activities. The greatest risk of transmitting Ebola virus is when symptoms first appear and are mild. Ebola rapidly progresses to severe disease that requires hospital care and ends social activities.

Chapter 5
Ebola Disease- through the Victim's Eyes

These are statements from patients who recovered from Ebola disease. This is how they felt and what they experienced during and after Ebola:

- I felt isolated and alone
- I was afraid I would never see my family again
- I was afraid my whole family would get the disease from me
- All I could see of my caregiver was his eyes behind the mask
- I was afraid I would give Ebola to my doctors and nurses
- I didn't feel like a person anymore- just a thing that no one wanted to be around
- I felt cut off from the land of the living
- I felt like a monster that everyone wanted to hide from
- I felt depersonalized
- I felt like my life was over
- I felt like I was floating away and would never return
- I felt like I had left the land of the living and was hovering above hell
- I felt like I was burning up
- I felt like no one cared about me and that I would die all alone
- I felt humiliated when I could not control my bodily functions
- I was terrified when I started vomiting blood

- I got progressively weaker until I didn't care if I lived or died
- I felt like a zombie. I couldn't move, I couldn't talk, I couldn't think. I didn't care.
- I prayed for the end to come quickly
- I had never been that sick or helpless before
- I recovered but I still feel weak and have muscle and joint pain
- I lived but I lost the spark that makes life worth living
- I beat Ebola
- I got a second chance and a new appreciation of what is really important in life
- I am too young to die
- I am not ready to die
- I knew I was dying
- I made peace with death
- I was ready to die so the pain would stop
- People who know I lived through Ebola look at me with fear and anxiety
- I feel ostracized by the people around me- no one wants to be with me
- I have become an object of pity and scorn
- I feel like I have been given a second chance at life
- God blessed me and I lived through Ebola disease

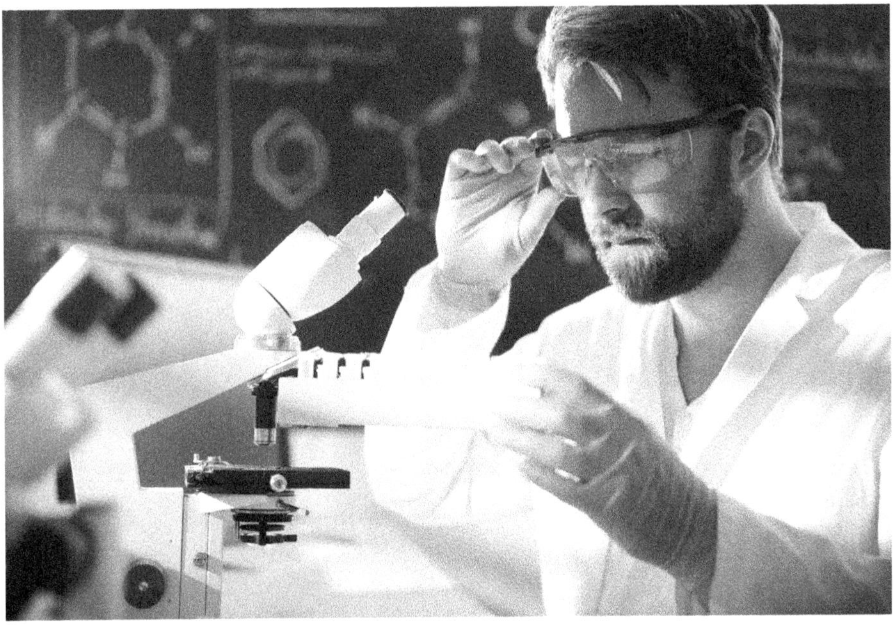

Part 2
Ebola Disease

Chapter 6
How Ebola Kills

Ebola is a filovirus. It belongs to a family of viruses called Filoviridae. There are five known strains of Ebola virus but only four are transmitted to humans. The 2014 Ebola pandemic is caused by the Zaire Ebolavirus which is the most virulent strain. It is classified as a level 4 bio-hazard by the CDC. Ebola virus contains one molecule of single-stranded, negative-sense RNA. It is curved into a distinctive u-shaped structure. Ebola survival is based on the survival of the animal or human host that it infects. The virus can only live outside of a living host for a few hours before it becomes inactive and incapable of causing Ebola disease.

Ebola virus is primarily transmitted by direct animal-to-human or human-to-human contact with the secretions of someone who has symptomatic Ebola disease and is shedding the virus. Ebola disease is considered a category 3 public health crisis of global magnitude. CDC and WHO guidelines and recommendations should be followed consistently and carefully.

Ebola virus enters the host after exposure to the blood or body fluids of a patient with symptomatic Ebola disease. The virus penetrates through mucus membranes, breaks in the skin, or puncture injuries with sharp medical instruments that are contaminated. Ebola infects many cell types including monocytes, macrophages, dendritic cells, endothelial cells, fibroblasts, hepatocytes, and adrenal cortical cells. Ebola virus migrates from the original infection site to regional lymph nodes- then to the liver, spleen, adrenal gland, and heart, brain, and kidneys.. Ebola infection turns the human body into a viral cloning factory that churns out massive numbers of Ebola virus particles. Ebola grows rapidly until the virus-damaged cell virtually explodes- releasing Ebola virus into healthy cells which also become infected. Every cell and organ of the body is affected. The immune system and Ebola fight for supremacy. When the immune systems wins- the patient recovers. When Ebola wins- the patient dies.

Ebola virus sends out chemicals that are released into the bloodstream. They stimulate the body's immune system. Many people infected with Ebola virus will be unable to develop an adequate immune response. Their immune system will be decimated and destroyed. About 60-90% of people who are infected with Ebola will die within one month.

- Ebola virus causes decreased white blood cell counts which leaves the patient susceptible to opportunistic infections. Antibiotics are ineffective against viruses.
- Ebola virus inactivates T-lymphocytes and decreases antibody production which compromises the victim's ability to mount an adequate immune response.
- Extensive organ damage occurs throughout victim's body resulting in multi-organ failure.
- Ebola virus reduces platelet counts and impairs normal blood clotting mechanisms. Uncontrolled bleeding, shock, and profuse hemorrhage occurs
- The most common causes of death from Ebola disease are multi-organ failure and uncontrollable bleeding. Infected people have organ failure, hemorrhage massively, and bleed out.

Chapter 7
Transmission

The carrier that caused the first Ebola outbreak in the Congo and Zaire in 1976 has never been identified. The CDC and WHO indicate that fruit bats carry Ebola virus and are indigenous to Western Africa. Infected bats may be responsible for transmission to other animals or humans who have contact with them. The number of different animals that can act as reservoirs for Ebola virus is not known. Antelopes and possums are known carriers of Ebola virus. Primates such as chimpanzees, apes, monkeys, and gorillas can be infected with Ebola disease and transmit Ebola virus.

Any animal that develops Ebola disease can infect other animals or humans who have contact with their secretions. Dead animal carcasses have a very high viral load and are extremely infectious. Large amounts of blood will be present on a dead animal's body- drawing scavengers who will be exposed to the Ebola virus and at risk of developing Ebola disease. Each infected animal can transmit Ebola disease to many others. The number of infected animals is unknown but increasing rapidly. The potential for transmitting Ebola virus from animals to humans is staggering.

Animal to human transmission rates are unknown but most African villagers hunt and trap animals. They use animal hides to make their clothing and they consume the meat as a major source of protein in their diet. Ebola infected animals will be ill and easy to trap and kill. Their blood and secretions will have high viral loads. The risk of Ebola disease among West African villagers is very high. The risk of Ebola disease spreading throughout the world is dependent on our ability to keep Ebola contained in Western Africa.

These are fundamental truths about the Ebola crisis of 2014:

- Ebola disease is wide-spread and under-reported in West African villages.
- Families are hiding their Ebola infected loved ones to keep them in the village with their family.
- Ebola disease is pandemic in Western Africa and it has spread into large population centers in Guinea, Liberia, Sierra Leone, and Mali.
- Porous country borders and easily accessible inter-continental flights will make it very hard to isolate and contain Ebola disease in Western Africa.
- The risk of Ebola disease spreading to other countries and nations of the world is increasing daily as the number of cases increase.
- It takes only one lapse in protective procedures to allow an Ebola infected traveler to leave Western Africa and bring the disease to other countries of the world.

The virus is spread by direct contact with the secretions of an infected animal or person. The virus can be shed in blood, saliva, vomit, feces, urine, sweat, semen, breast milk, and vaginal secretions. People are infectious as long as their blood and body fluids are shedding virus. The WHO indicates that men can shed the virus in semen for as long as 7 weeks after recovery from Ebola disease. Men who have recovered from Ebola disease should abstain from sexual relations for three months past recovery.

The people at greatest risk of getting Ebola disease are those who are caring for patients infected with Ebola. That includes family members, health care workers, laboratory personnel, morticians, pathologists, funeral directors, surgeons, and people responsible for laundering and sterilizing supplies. Close surveillance for signs of illness, early diagnosis, and appropriate treatment are critical to reduce transmission of Ebola virus.

Used needles, soiled linens, and contaminated medical equipment can also shed virus and cause Ebola disease. Any surface that is contaminated with blood or body secretions that contain Ebola virus can act as a vector. Estimates by the CDC and WHO indicate they can cause infection for about 24 hours but the chance of infection is dramatically reduced after the first few hours.

The bodies of humans who die of Ebola disease are very contagious. There is usually a lot of blood and body secretions on the bodies and viral shedding is very high. The CDC has very specific recommendations for burials of people who die of Ebola disease.

Ebola is not an airborne disease. The virus does not float in the air and it is not spread by breathing. It is not spread through water or food. Transmission requires contact with the secretions of an infected animal or person. Broken skin surfaces and improper use of personal protective equipment increases the risk of transmission.

A patient must have symptoms to spread the disease to others. Anyone who has been **exposed to an animal or person with Ebola disease and has not developed symptoms within 21 days is not infected and will not become sick with Ebola.**

Anyone who recovers from Ebola disease and is symptom free does not have the disease and is not shedding the virus. They can lead a normal life. Survivors of Ebola disease have antibodies against Ebola virus and will have natural immunity for up to ten years.

Chapter 8
Signs and Symptoms

Exposure to Ebola virus occurs when someone has direct contact with the secretions of an animal or person who has Ebola disease. The virus enters the bloodstream and begins to spread and infect cells.

The **incubation period** is the amount of time from exposure to the virus until symptoms develop. When symptoms are present- a person has active disease and is shedding the virus. They can infect others and should be isolated to prevent transmission of the virus.

The incubation for Ebola disease is 2-21 days. People usually show symptoms about 8- 10 days after exposure to the virus. **The Ebola virus can only be shed by someone who has Ebola disease and is sick. Someone who had exposure but has not developed symptoms within 21 days does not have the disease and cannot shed the virus.**

- Early signs of the disease include:
- Sudden onset of high fever (greater than 101.5 degrees)
- Severe headache
- Muscle pain
- Extreme weakness
- Malaise
- Joint pain
- Sore throat
- Lack of appetite

Late symptoms of Ebola disease start about 3-6 days after the onset of symptoms and are progressive:

- Persistent Vomiting
- Profuse diarrhea
- Stomach pain
- Abdominal pain
- Rash
- Bruising
- Chest pain
- Shortness of breath
- Organ damage of the liver and kidneys
- Unexplained bruising
- End stage organ failure
- Shock
- Hemorrhage- severe and uncontrollable
- Seizures
- Confusion
- Coma
- Death

Patients presenting with early Ebola disease have symptoms that are typical of any viral illness. Other viruses and diseases that could present with the same symptoms include influenza, MERS, encephalitis, avian flu, Dengue fever, meningitis, yellow fever, West Nile virus, malaria, cholera, and hepatitis. People who are ill and being screened for Ebola disease need to be thoroughly screened for all of these other diseases to accurately diagnose the cause of their illness.

influenza cases present with symptoms that are similar to early Ebola disease but there are important distinctions that differentiate influenza from Ebola disease.

Influenza:

- Respiratory illness caused by a flu virus.
- Airborne disease that is spread by droplets secreted by coughing, sneezing, and talking.
- Viral particles are found on surfaces but this is an uncommon form of transmission.
- Anyone can get influenza.
- Children, the elderly, and immuno-compromised people are at greatest risk of serious complications including death.
- Incubation period is 2 days.
- Produces mild to moderate illness and recovery for most is within one week.
- Other symptoms that are rarely seen in Ebola include cough and nasal congestion.

Ebola disease:

- Rare and deadly.
- Caused by infection by the Ebola virus.
- Spread by direct contact with blood or body fluids of an infected animal or person.
- Spread by direct contact with the dead body of someone who died of Ebola.
- Contaminated needles, medical supplies, or linen can be sources of infection if body fluids are present.
- Greatest risk of Ebola disease is in people who are caring for family members with Ebola disease and health care workers who care for patients with Ebola disease.
- People who have travelled to Ebola infected countries are at risk of exposure.
- Incubation period is 2- 21 days- the average time for onset of symptoms is 8-10 days.
- Symptoms start with mild symptoms that get progressively worse.

- Ebola disease lasts up to a month and 60-90% die as a result of the disease.
- **People do not spread the Ebola virus until symptoms appear**.
- Patients with advanced Ebola disease are very sick and it is obvious that they do not have influenza.

Chapter 9
Diagnosis

A diagnosis of Ebola disease requires thorough medical evaluation by a qualified clinician. Three main risk factors should be considered when making a diagnosis of Ebola disease.

- Identify **exposure history:** Has the patient lived in or travelled to a country with widespread Ebola transmission or high rates of disease? Have they had contact with any individual with confirmed Ebola disease in the last 21 days? Did they have contact with the secretions of an infected person? Did they use personal protective equipment?
- Identify **signs and symptoms**: Do they have fever? What other symptoms do they have that are characteristic of Ebola disease? What is the severity of the illness? How many days has it been since the last exposure to someone with Ebola disease?
- Obtain **laboratory specimens** for definitive diagnosis of Ebola disease.

Ebola can be detected in the blood after symptoms of Ebola disease appear. It may take up to three days to have detectible levels of the virus in the blood. If a patient has had exposure to Ebola virus and has a negative blood test- they should be retested in 3 days. Any specimens that are obtained and sent out for confirmatory testing need to be triple packed in a durable and leak proof container and transported according to CDC recommendations.

Anyone who has been exposed to Ebola virus and has symptoms of Ebola disease needs to be isolated and quarantined until the diagnosis is confirmed or rejected. Personal protective equipment should be used by all people who have contact with them. All suspected cases need to be reported to the infection control department of the hospital and the local and state public health departments. When Ebola disease is confirmed by laboratory testing- the CDC must be notified. Family members and those who have had direct contact with a patient with confirmed Ebola disease should be quarantined for 21 days past the time of exposure.

Suspicious laboratory findings are usually identified on routine blood tests that are done on admission to a hospital. These are some expected findings:

- WBCs are decreased with a shift to the left, neutrophils are increased
- Platelets are decreased
- Amylase is elevated
- ALT/AST are elevated
- Proteinuria is present
- PT and PTT are elevated, Fibrinogen is decreased

Laboratory tests are available to diagnose Ebola disease. Blood specimens detect specific antigens and genes of the virus. Testing for Ebola disease is done by a CLIA compliant lab using the highest biohazard safety precautions. The lab must comply with all CDC regulations and guidelines.

Some of the tests that are available for Ebola virus diagnosis are:

- RT-PCR (reverse transcriptase polymerase chain reaction)- suspected Ebola virus is observed for replication and the results are analyzed by electrophoresis.
- ELISA (enzyme-linked immunosorbant assay)–this test is an antibody capture test that detects the presence of Ebola virus by producing a color change when Ebola virus reacts to the patient's serum.
- Immuno-fluorescent assay can be performed by microscopic evaluation of a single layer of cells fixed on a slide. The results are confirmed using a western blot procedure.
- IgG or IgM- specific immunoglobulin assays can be performed to diagnose Ebola disease.

- Electron microscopy can detect the Ebola virus. This test does not have the specificity or sensitivity of some of the other diagnostic tests.
- Ebola virus can be isolated from cell cultures.

People under investigation (PUI) for Ebola have significant exposure histories and present to the hospital for evaluation with symptoms that indicate increased risk of Ebola disease. People become confirmed cases when confirmatory lab tests are positive for Ebola disease.

Patients who have recovered from Ebola disease will continue to have positive IgM and IgG antibodies. Someone who had Ebola exposure and died suspiciously without being tested can still be diagnosed by using RT-PCR analysis.

There are newer non-invasive diagnostic tests that are being field tested in Western Africa where Ebola disease rates are high. They involve testing urine and saliva samples. The tests do not have to be sent out to other labs and the risk of exposure to Ebola virus from contaminated needles is eliminated. The results are available more rapidly so decisions can be made quickly about the need for family or community quarantine. The goal of diagnosing Ebola disease is always to isolate cases, quarantine people who are at risk, and prevent the spread of Ebola disease to non-infected people.

Chapter 10
Treatment

Ebola disease treatment is non-specific. Our sophisticated, high-tech medical system has no definitive answer for how to manage Ebola disease. The treatment we give is ineffective in about 60- 90% of cases.

- There are no antiviral medications that treat Ebola disease.
- Antibiotics are ineffective against Ebola disease.
- There is no cure for Ebola disease.
- There are no FDA-approved vaccines to prevent Ebola disease although several are under investigation.

Supportive care is the only current treatment for a patient with Ebola disease. The goal is to help the patient develop an adequate antibody response and support his body's efforts to heal. The strength of his immune system is directly linked to his chance of recovery.

Most patients infected with Ebola disease will need to be hospitalized- the majority will be in intensive care. Infection control measures are the cornerstone of preventing the spread of Ebola virus. The infectious diseases department in the hospital should be involved in every Ebola patient's care and the local and state public health departments should be notified about their admission. Community assessment for exposure risk and quarantine necessity should be conducted by the public health officials. Any confirmed case of Ebola disease must be reported to the CDC.

Any patient with Ebola disease should be isolated in a single patient room with a private bathroom. The door should be closed at all times. A log book should be kept to document the names of all people who entered the patient's room and the function they performed. The patient's care should be given by a small group of care providers. No one else should have access to the room and PPE should be used correctly and consistently.

Visitors should be strictly limited to people that are critical to the patient's well-being. Any family member who stays with their loved one must use personal protective equipment (PPE) and should be in quarantine until 21 days after the exposure ends.

Hand-washing and other infection control measures should be used consistently to avoid disease spread to other patients or health care workers. Personal protective equipment must be used at all times by all healthcare workers who are caring for Ebola patients. Proper handling and disposal of contaminated medical supplies is critical. Disposable medical equipment should be used whenever possible. Non-disposable medical equipment should be cleaned and disinfected according to the manufacturer's instructions, hospital policies, and CDC guidelines.

Supportive care of patients with Ebola disease improves survival rates. Symptoms are identified and treated as they occur. Treatment is designed to slow the progression of the disease and support the immune system of the patient. These are some of the treatments that are being used to treat Ebola patients:

- Intravenous fluids for rehydration
- Electrolyte replacement
- Parenteral nutrition
- Pain control
- Oxygen if oxygen saturation levels are low
- Antibiotics if there are signs of opportunistic infection
- Vasopressors to maintain blood pressure and perfusion when septic shock is present
- Transfusions of platelets or whole blood for shock, hemorrhage, or disseminated intravascular coagulation (DIC)

Despite the care that is given to patients with Ebola disease- large numbers will die. Extreme care must be taken when handling the bodies of patients who have died of Ebola disease. Dead bodies shed large amounts of active

Ebola virus and are capable of infecting other people. Personnel who work in morgues or mortuaries are also at significant risk of infection with Ebola virus and should use PPE, common sense, and caution.

Chapter 11

Unapproved Investigational Treatments

The United States Food and Drug Administration (FDA) is the governmental agency that regulates drug therapies that are approved for use in the United States. Currently- there is no FDA approved vaccine to prevent Ebola disease and no FDA approved drug to treat Ebola disease.

Several drugs for "investigational use only" were used on very small numbers of patients with Ebola disease in Western Africa. The results were considered promising. More research is needed to determine safety and efficacy. Larger case numbers will be needed to meet the guidelines for FDA approval. The United States government is funding grants and research projects to evaluate drugs rapidly and to bring effective treatments and drugs to the marketplace. Effective vaccines and drugs are desperately needed in Western Africa now.

A WHO advisory panel was convened to consider and assess ethical implications and clinical decision making about using unregistered interventions that showed promising results in the laboratory or on animal models but had not been evaluated for safety and efficacy in humans. The panel concluded unanimously that their use was acceptable on ethical and evidentiary grounds provided certain conditions were met:

- There was general acknowledgment that this therapy was a departure from our well-established and historically evolved system of regulation and governance of therapies and interventions approved for use.
- Any investigational use of unapproved therapies must provide transparency about all aspects of care.

- The goal was to generate the maximal amount of knowledge and data on the effects of the intervention.
- There was to be a fair decision process about who would have access to the treatment since the number of doses available for use was very limited.
- There would be universal acceptance and agreement about the process used.
- The patient would receive full informed consent.
- The patient had the right to choose whether to use the therapy or not.
- Complete confidentiality was required.
- The patient would be treated with respect and dignity.
- There would be some degree of community oversight of the process.

Zmapp is the drug that was used in Western Africa on a very small number of cases of Ebola disease. There was only enough Zmapp produced to treat seven patients. Two patients with advanced disease died but Zmapp showed promising results. Additional quantities are being produced for a larger "investigational use" study in Western Africa. Zmapp is a monoclonal antibody that attaches to the surface of Ebola virus and neutralizes its activity. Zmapp is still in clinical trials and has not been approved for use by the FDA.

Blood transfusions using donated blood from recovered Ebola victims has also been used in Western Africa to treat Ebola patients. Anyone who recovers from Ebola disease has protective antibodies that will prevent Ebola disease for up to ten years. These are the research questions that we are trying to answer: Can using transfused blood from recovered victims give passive antibodies to an Ebola patient? Can it stop the disease or slow its progression? Can it increase survival rates or decrease the severity of the disease? The results of this therapy have been mixed and no conclusions have been reached about the efficacy of this treatment for Ebola disease.

This is where we are now in our efforts to cure or prevent Ebola disease:

- No antiviral medications for treatment.
- No FDA approved drug regimen for treatment.

- No cure.
- No vaccine.
- 60-90% mortality rate.

Standard Ebola treatment in the United States and the world continues to be supportive care. The patient is still fighting Ebola using his compromised immune system- while researchers continue to work to find a vaccine, to find a cure, and to find an effective treatment.

Chapter 12
Prevention

Ebola disease is pandemic in Western Africa in 2014 but very few cases have been reported outside of Africa. The key to preventing Ebola disease from spreading globally is to contain Ebola virus in Africa and break the chain of transmission within the West African countries with widespread disease.

Controlling the pandemic in West Africa will require:

- Learning to avoid practices and behaviors that increase the risk of Ebola exposure and disease.
- Education of all African citizens about how Ebola virus is transmitted and how to protect their families and communities.
- Teaching the importance of hygiene, clean homes, and good health practices in preventing Ebola disease.
- Teaching epidemic control measures including isolation, contact identification, and quarantine.
- Encouraging the use of soap and water, alcohol-based hand sanitizers, detergents, disinfectants, and household bleach to prevent Ebola virus transmission.
- Encourage frequent hand washing.
- Decreasing the risk of animal-to-human transmission from contact with infected bats or primates or handling dead animals. Animals should only be handled using gloves and protective clothing. Bush meat should never be handled without gloves or

consumed raw. All meat should be thoroughly cooked before eating.

- Decreasing human-to-human transmission which usually occurs as a result of direct contact with infectious blood or body secretions of someone with symptomatic Ebola disease.
- CDC disease detectives and humanitarian aid workers in remote villages of the bush looking for high-risk populations and identifying people with Ebola virus exposure and disease.
- Identifying people in cities with exposure to Ebola virus and monitoring their movement for 21 days past their last exposure.
- Case identification of **every person** with Ebola disease.
- Contact tracing of anyone exposed to someone with symptomatic Ebola disease.
- Isolation of every contact for 21 days after their last exposure.
- Quarantine of families and communities with exposure to symptomatic Ebola patients.
- Laboratory services capable of rapid and accurate diagnosis of Ebola disease.
- Ebola treatment units and community care centers staffed with adequate personnel, medical equipment, and supplies.
- Medical personnel who are highly trained in caring for Ebola patients and are able to use PPE correctly and consistently.
- Specific procedures to handle the blood and body fluids of patients with Ebola disease- including safe laboratory specimen collection and safe injection practices.
- Appropriate procedures for handling the dead bodies of Ebola victims.
- Burial teams that are able to provide culturally sensitive and safe burials of victims of Ebola disease in Western Africa.
- Knowledge of appropriate cleaning, disinfection, and decontamination procedures that should be followed wherever Ebola patients are being cared for or have died.

- Exit screening procedures and monitoring and movement protocols that will prevent people with exposure to Ebola virus or symptoms of Ebola disease from getting on commercial airlines and going to other parts of the world that do not have widespread Ebola disease.
- Appropriate guarding and closure of the borders of African nations with widespread disease to prevent exposed or infected people from leaving the country on foot or by car.
- The commitment and cooperation of every nation in the world to provide financial resources and medical assistance to countries of Western Africa who have widespread Ebola disease.

The risk of widespread Ebola disease in the United States is very low. Citizens are at greater risk of being infected by influenza than Ebola disease. Americans should take reasonable precautions but should not give in to feelings of fear, hopelessness, or panic. These are some general guidelines to reduce the risk of being exposed to any infectious disease, including Ebola:

- Wash your hands frequently with soap and water or alcohol-based hand sanitizer.
- Encourage anyone who is coughing and sneezing to cover their mouth and nose.
- Use a plastic bag for disposal of used tissues or air sick bags.
- Do not share personal care items like toothbrushes or hair care items.
- Do surface cleaning of counters, shelves, and appliances with disinfectants daily.
- Sanitize sinks, toilets, and showers regularly.
- Practice safe cooking habits.
- Do not share drinking glasses or eating utensils.
- Use your dishwasher to sanitize your dishes at high temperatures.
- Avoid large crowds.
- Do not engage in social activities during large outbreaks of infectious disease.
- Practice safe sex.

- Use caution around animals you don't know. Avoid handling animal secretions.
- Be cautious and alert in all areas of your life to avoid infectious exposures or physical injuries.

Our government, the CDC, and the public health system have established procedures, protocols, guidelines, and recommendation that are designed to keep Ebola from entering America. Every case of Ebola disease in the United States has been from one of these three categories:

- People infected during travel to West African countries with widespread Ebola disease.
- Healthcare workers who took care of patients with Ebola disease.
- Humanitarian aid workers who gave aid in Western Africa and were air-flighted back to the United States for emergency medical care.

The United States has one of the best health care systems in the world. Patients who have Ebola disease will get state-of-the-art care by well-trained personnel using rigorous infection control measures. People with Ebola virus exposure and contacts of patients with Ebola disease are being evaluated and actively monitored by the public health authorities daily for up to 21 days past their last exposure. Everyone who has Ebola disease and all of their contacts are known and being followed carefully.

The procedures and policies of the CDC and the public health authorities will be reviewed in the next section of the book. Their guidelines and recommendations are designed to prevent widespread Ebola disease in the United States. They also provide a framework for managing people with exposure to Ebola virus or patients with Ebola disease.

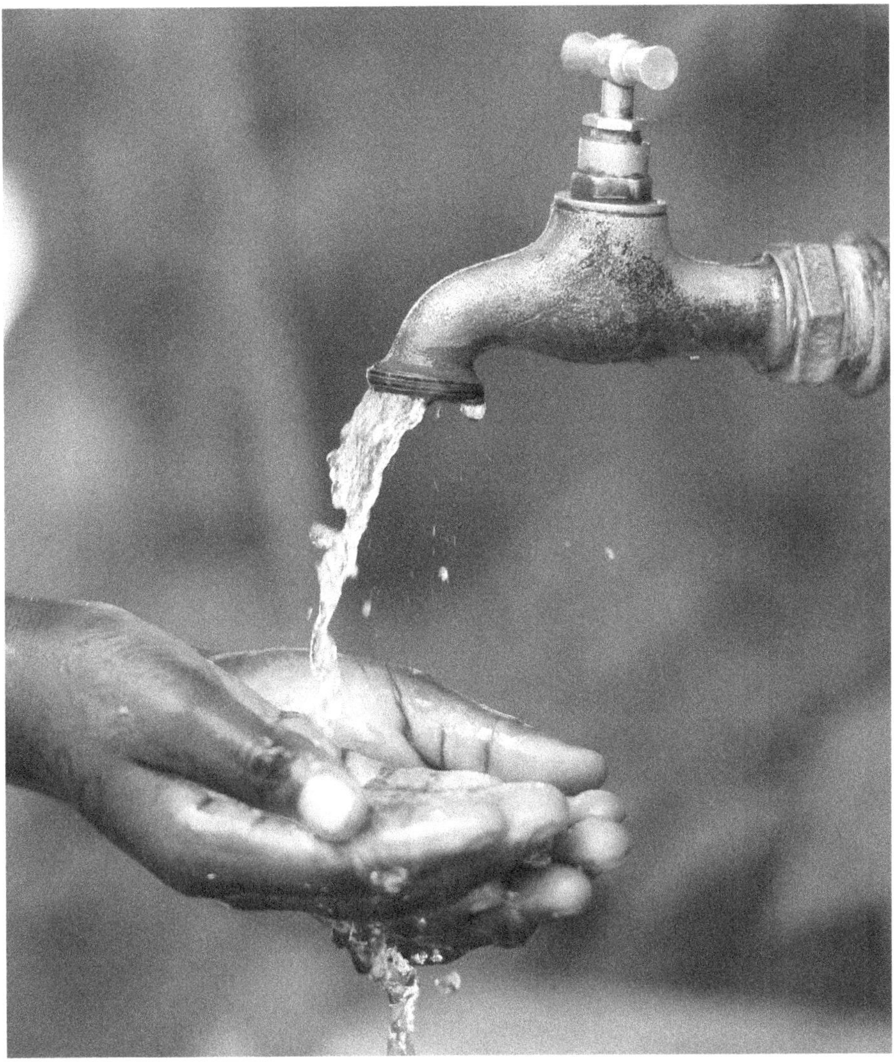

Part 3
Ebola Guidelines and Recommendations

Chapter 13
The CDC's Role

WESTERN AFRICA: CDC's action plan and response to the ongoing crisis:

The Center for Disease Control has activated its Emergency Operations Center (EOC) to help co-ordinate ongoing relief efforts in Western Africa in partnership with other health and humanitarian organizations. Widespread Ebola disease is affecting multiple countries in and around Western Africa. The CDC has sent teams of public health experts to assess and evaluate the situation. They have more than 100 disease detectives on the ground in Western Africa. The CDC is providing technical expertise and tactical support in co-operation with governments and health care systems from around the world. The goal of the international effort is to keep Ebola disease from spreading globally to other continents and countries.

The CDC brings unparalleled knowledge about how Ebola spreads, how it kills, how to find it, and how to stop it. The CDC is working in co-operation with The World Health Organization (WHO) and many international agencies and emergency response experts. A massive relief operation is underway- but more help is needed and time is of the essence.

The Emergency Operations Center is functioning at level 1, its highest level, because of the significance and threat to the world from the 2014 Ebola pandemic in Western Africa. The EOC can be called to report confirmed cases of Ebola disease or for consultation at (770)-488-7100.

- CDC's disease detectives are finding and investigating emerging cases, they are identifying contacts of people with Ebola disease, and they are assessing the need for family and community quarantines. They are working in the bush and in remote villages where Ebola disease is wide-spread. Their goal is to find the sick, isolate anyone who has been exposed, and prevent Ebola virus from spreading to healthy people.

- CDC's scientists in the lab are diagnosing Ebola cases. They are also cracking the codes of Ebola's DNA to map outbreak connections and links.
- CDC's outbreak control specialists are identifying patterns of spread and areas of population that are the most vulnerable so that scarce resources can be deployed where the need is greatest.
- CDC's Ebola outbreak veterans are leading the way with expert guidance and support to national and international agencies involved in the relief efforts and new recruits joining the Ebola fight.
- CDC's communication specialists are dispersing information about Ebola disease and teaching how to avoid exposure and infection. They are using mass media reports, press releases, fact sheets, and daily advisories. They are involved in ongoing on-the-ground activities. They are working every day to discourage rumors, stigmatization, and unsafe practices. They are telling the real story about Ebola disease using real statistics and knowledge gained from studying characteristics of the 2014 Ebola epidemic.
- CDC's emergency operations teams bring incident management expertise to the team and are evaluating complex situations and making critical decisions in the ongoing crisis.

UNITED STATES OF AMERICA: CDC's action plan and response

In the United States- the CDC has established protocols, guidelines, and recommendations to protect American citizens. CDC is working in co-operation with many organizations in the United States to ensure safe airline arrivals and to secure borders that act as entry points into the United States. Many other organizations have critical roles in ensuring that Ebola disease does not threaten people who live in the United States. The Department of Homeland Security, Department of Defense, Department of Health and Human Services, Department of Naturalization and Immigration, Department of Customs and Border Patrol, and the National Public Health

Department are all actively involved in the efforts and are working in co-operation with the CDC to keep Americans safe and healthy.

The risk of Ebola disease in the United States is very low. Only health care workers who have cared for patients with symptomatic Ebola disease have been infected while they were in the United States. Despite the low risk of Ebola virus transmission in the United States and the low number of cases of Ebola disease- our government, the CDC, our national public health system and our medical care system are vigilant and ready to care for anyone in the United States who has been exposed to Ebola virus or has Ebola disease.

The CDC has been active in protecting Americans by providing leadership, information, and expertise. These are some of the policies, guidelines, and actions that the CDC has taken to help keep Ebola disease out of America. The CDC:

- Maintains an up-to-date and comprehensive website that keeps people on the cutting-edge of developments related to Ebola disease. It gives updated statistics and information in near real-time. CDC policies, protocols, guidelines, recommendations, and updates are available as soon as events unfold in the field.
- Has established guidelines for classifying exposure risk.
- Has established a protocol for enhanced screening of people with Ebola exposure. It includes monitoring and movement restrictions for anyone with exposure to Ebola virus or symptoms of Ebola disease.
- Gives recommendations for safe travel to Western Africa.
- Sets protocols and gives guidelines for screening travelers returning to the United States from any international destination including Western Africa.
- Provides training for health care workers on infection control and how to use PPE correctly.
- Receives reports and monitors all cases of Ebola disease in the United States.
- Provides state-of-the art lab facilities that are involved in testing specimens of people with suspected Ebola disease.

- Works actively with the public health system to ensure that all people with Ebola exposure or disease are known and being actively monitored.
- Sets the standards for safe patient triage in homes, communities, and hospitals.
- Encourages innovative therapies and techniques such as whole genome sequencing and analysis, monitoring for mutation patterns and changes related to Ebola transmission, re-designing personal protective equipment to make it safer and more comfortable.
- Supports research to find a vaccine for prevention of Ebola disease and encourages agencies that are conducting vaccine trials to prove safety and efficacy.
- The CDC Foundation is providing critical assistance and supplies through donations to the CDC Foundation's Global Disaster Response Fund.

The CDC is active and involved in the West African bush and on the home front- working to eradicate Ebola and to triage and treat its victims. The CDC is working tirelessly to help the West African nations who are in the midst of the biggest health crisis the world has ever seen. They are our guardians at the gate in the United States- keeping us safe and standing guard against Ebola disease.

Chapter 14
Exposure Risk Classification

Many epidemiologic risk factors need to be considered when evaluating a person who has had Ebola exposure. Placing people with Ebola exposure into risk categories allow reasonable decisions to be made about whether monitoring and movement restrictions are warranted. It also aids in decision-making about the need for contact identification and quarantine.

"High risk" exposures include any of the following

- Percutaneous (needle sticks) or mucous membrane (broken skin and open sores) exposure involving the blood or body fluids of a person with Ebola disease while he was symptomatic.
- Exposure to the blood or body fluids of a person with Ebola disease without personal protective equipment (PPE) while he/she was symptomatic. Body fluids would include but not be limited to: blood, feces, vomit, saliva, sweat, tears, urine, semen, vaginal secretions, and breast milk.
- Processing the blood or body fluids of a patient with known Ebola disease without using appropriate PPE and biosafety precautions. Examples would be laboratory specimen collections, biopsies, or autopsy.
- Direct contact with a dead body without appropriate PPE in a country with widespread Ebola virus transmission (Guinea, Liberia, Sierra Leone, or Mali).
- Any person who gave direct care to someone with Ebola disease without using appropriate PPE while the patient was symptomatic.

- Any person who was living in the immediate household of someone with Ebola disease while he was symptomatic.

"Some risk" exposures include any of the following behaviors when traveling to countries with widespread Ebola virus transmission such as Guinea, Liberia, Sierra Leone, or Mali

- Direct contact with a person who has Ebola disease and is symptomatic while using PPE.
- Direct contact with the body fluids of a person who has Ebola disease and is symptomatic while using PPE.
- Close contact with a patient with Ebola disease while they were symptomatic. The location of the contact can be the household, hospital, or community. Close contact is defined as being exposed for a prolonged period of time while not wearing PPE and being within a distance of approximately 3 feet of a person who is symptomatic.

"Low but not zero risk" exposures include any of the following

- Having been in a country with widespread Ebola virus transmission (Guinea, Libya, Sierra Leone, or Mali) within the last 21 days but having no known exposure.
- Having brief direct contact such as shaking hands or touching while not wearing appropriate PPE with a person who was in the early stages of Ebola disease.
- Brief proximity with a person with Ebola disease while that person was symptomatic.
- Direct contact using appropriate PPE with a person who does not live in Guinea, Liberia, Sierra Leone, or Mali but who has Ebola disease and is symptomatic.
- Someone who travelled on an aircraft with a person with Ebola disease while that person was symptomatic.

"No identifiable risk" includes

- Contact with an asymptomatic person who had exposure to a person with Ebola disease.

- Contact with a person who developed Ebola disease before they had symptoms.
- Elapsed time of greater than 21 days after returning from a country with widespread Ebola virus transmission such as Guinea, Liberia, Sierra Leone, or Mali.
- Travel to any country in Africa except Guinea, Liberia, Sierra Leone, or Mali with no exposures as listed above.
- Aircraft or ship crew members who remain on or in immediate proximity to the airplane or ship and have no direct contact with anyone of the community during the entire time that the conveyance is present in any country with widespread Ebola virus transmission such as Guinea, Libya, Sierra Leone, or Mali.

Knowing the type of exposure a person had to Ebola virus helps authorities to determine his risk of developing symptomatic Ebola disease. It is also used to decide whether he needs monitoring and movement restrictions or other public health interventions.

Chapter 15
Enhanced Screening Protocol

The CDC has established monitoring and movement protocols for travelers returning to the United States from the West African countries of Guinea, Liberia, Sierra Leone, and Mali. These guidelines also apply to travelers from any foreign country whose routes included stops in Western Africa. Any person with exposure to Ebola virus or contact with the secretions of someone with known Ebola disease will be monitored using the enhanced screening protocol.

The Department of Homeland Security (DHS) and the Center for Disease Control (CDC) have designated five major airport hubs in the United States as entry points for flights originating from Western Africa. These airports are JFK Airport in New York, Newark Airport in New Jersey, Dulles Airport in Washington DC, O'Hare Airport in Chicago, and Hartsville-Jackson Airport in Atlanta. Using these major hubs as entry points for high risk flights and using enhanced screening techniques are predicted to successfully screen over 94% of travelers returning from the affected countries.

The goal of enhanced screening is to look for sick travelers with any contagious diseases- including but not limited to Ebola disease. Airport staff is trained to investigate any reports of sick travelers and triage them appropriately using the CDC guidelines. The public health system is also involved in the enhanced screening protocol and will take an active role in assessing and managing people at risk of Ebola disease in their homes and communities. Current CDC guidelines recommend direct active monitoring by the public health department of all people who have had exposure to Ebola virus. Self-monitoring is not recommended.

These are the basic components of the enhanced screening protocol for travelers returning from affected areas or any passengers suspected of having potentially infectious diseases:

- Each passenger at risk will receive a CARE kit that includes a thermometer, symptom card, and log book to enter the results of the daily health checks for 21 days past the last potential exposure to Ebola virus.
- Temperature will be taken twice a day- in the morning and evening.
- Daily symptom checks will look for fever, headache, muscle or joint pain, increased fatigue or weakness, vomiting, diarrhea, stomach pain, or unusual bruising or bleeding.
- A public health worker will come to your home for direct assessment of your condition once a day if you are considered at high risk and in need of direct active monitoring by the public health department.
- A public healthcare worker will contact you once or twice a day for active monitoring if your assessed level of risk requires public health assessment. They will review your temperature, symptoms, and general health.
- If you have any symptoms- you must follow the recommendations of the public health care worker who contacts you.
- If you have had exposure to Ebola virus and you have symptoms- do not be afraid. Seek medical care to protect yourself, your family, and your community.
- If someone with Ebola virus exposure becomes very sick- call 911 and the hospital. Warn them about the Ebola exposure so they are ready to take appropriate infection control precautions and so they can plan for appropriate triage and care in the Emergency Room.

The enhanced screening protocol makes public health authorities aware of every patient who has Ebola disease in the United States of America. The local public health department will be involved in screening his family and contacts and assessing their risk of Ebola. The public health department and CDC will decide on appropriate interventions for families and communities of patients with exposure to Ebola virus or confirmed Ebola disease.

Chapter 16
Hand Hygiene

Ebola virus is transmitted to healthy people when they come into direct contact with the blood or body fluids of symptomatic animals or people who have Ebola disease. The virus enters the body through:

- Cuts and abrasions of the skin.
- Exposed mucous membranes of the mouth, nose, and eyes.
- Puncture of the skin by contaminated needles or sharp instruments.

Our hands are our weakest link and the most common cause of infectious exposures. Hand hygiene is your first line of defense in protecting yourself from Ebola virus.

When should hand hygiene be done?

- Before touching a patient. Hand washing should be done before shaking hands or assisting in personal care activities such as moving him or helping him bathe. Any time you touch him to give him care, whether invasive or non-invasive, hand hygiene is a critical component of infection control.
- Before any clean or aseptic procedure you need to perform for him. Examples would be brushing his teeth, putting in eye drops, performing a rectal exam, inserting a suppository, giving an injection, dressing a wound, or inserting an invasive medical device such as a catheter, or nasogastric tube.
- Before putting on PPE and after taking off PPE.

- After exposure to blood or body fluids. Exposures can happen as a result of needle sticks or splashes with infectious body fluids. Failure to use PPE consistently or correctly increases the risk of exposure. Procedures such as drawing blood samples, removing medical devices, and changing dressings can result in unanticipated exposure to infectious diseases.
- After touching a patient. Whenever you complete your care of a patient and are ready to leave the room- wash your hands. When you are outside of his room- wash them again.
- After touching the patient's surroundings. Surfaces are easily contaminated with the patient's germs and secretions. Activities such as changing bed linens, cleaning bedside furniture, touching buttons on alarms or monitors can be sources of exposure to infectious agents. Hand hygiene protects you from germs on your hands and keeps you from spreading germs to other areas of the health care environment.

How should hand hygiene be done?

Soap and water should always be used when the hands are visibly soiled. Soap and water is considered the gold standard of hand hygiene and the best way to remove infectious organisms from your skin.

- Wet your hands with clean, running water- either hot or cold.
- Apply enough soap to cover all hand surfaces.
- Rub your hands palm to palm.
- Rub the back of your hands by using the palm of the opposite hand.
- Interlace the fingers and clean all finger surfaces.
- Clasp the thumb in the opposite closed palm and rub the thumb in a rotational manner.
- Scrub your hands for at least 40-60 seconds.
- Rinse your hands well under clean, running water.
- Dry your hands thoroughly using a clean dry single-use towel.
- Use the towel to turn off the water.
- Your hands are clean.

Alcohol-based hand sanitizers can be used when soap and water is not available. Hand sanitizers are not as effective when the hands or visibly soiled or greasy.

- Apply enough sanitizer to your cupped hand to cover all surfaces of the hands.
- Rub your hands palm to palm.
- Rub the back of your hands by using the palm of the opposite hand.
- Interlace the fingers and clean all finger surfaces.
- Clasp the thumb in the opposite closed palm and rub the thumb in a rotational manner.
- Rub your hands for at least 20-30 seconds until they are thoroughly dry.
- Your hands are clean.

Other times to use hand hygiene

- Before, during, and after preparing food.
- Before eating food.
- After using the toilet.
- Before and after changing diapers or cleaning up a child who has used the toilet.
- After blowing your nose, coughing, or sneezing.
- After personal grooming like brushing teeth, combing hair, or shaving.
- After touching an animal, animal food, or animal waste.
- After handling pet food or pet treats.
- After touching garbage.

Keeping your hands clean and free of infectious organisms is the easiest way to ensure your health and keep your family safe. Hand washing is the best and most effective way to protect the ones you love from Ebola disease. Be sure that you always have alcohol-based hand sanitizers and tissues with you when you leave your home. Use them liberally and offer them to everyone around you.

Chapter 17
Personal Protective Equipment

Personal protective equipment (PPE) acts as a barrier between the wearer and the work environment. It keeps potentially harmful or infectious organisms from direct contact with someone who could become infected.

Exposure to the infected blood or body fluids of a patient with symptomatic Ebola disease allows transmission of Ebola virus to healthy people. When PPE is used correctly and consistently it acts as a shield of protection that blocks Ebola virus transmission.

The CDC has set strict guidelines for the use of PPE in the United States health care system. There may be small variations in the guidelines used in other countries or in Western Africa but these guidelines should be fairly representative.

Any medical personnel who will be involved in the care of a patient with Ebola disease should have had a very intensive training course on the proper use of PPE. They must have performed frequent repetitions of witnessed drills and demonstrated correct technique while putting on and taking off PPE. They must have competency in performing all Ebola-related infection control procedures.

These are basic principles of correct PPE usage:

- PPE must be put on correctly in the proper order before entering the patient care environment.
- No adjustments to the PPE should be made in the patient care area.
- All skin must be covered before entering the patient care area
- PPE should remain in place and be worn correctly for the duration of exposure to the contaminated patient care environment.
- Healthcare workers should perform frequent disinfection of contaminated outer gloves using alcohol-based hand sanitizers-especially when handling body fluids.

- If there is any accidental breach in PPE procedure- the healthcare worker should go to the area where PPE is removed to assess the exposure and implement the facility exposure plan.
- Removing used PPE is a high-risk process that requires a structured procedure, a trained observer, and a designated area for safe removal.
- PPE should be removed slowly, carefully, and in the right sequence to decrease the possibility of self-contamination or other exposure to Ebola virus.
- A consistent process should be used in all training and competency drills to ensure that the same sequence is used by all staff and that breaches in the process are quickly identified.
- Trained observers should be witnesses every time a healthcare worker puts on or takes off PPE. Observers should read aloud each step in the procedure checklist then visually confirm and document that the step was performed correctly.

Any facility that cares for Ebola patients should ensure that there is adequate space and that the layout of the care area allows for clear separation between clean and contaminated areas. There should be a one-way flow of care from clean areas (where PPE is put on and preparation is made to enter the patient care environment) to contaminated areas (where healthcare workers exit from the patient care environment and remove PPE). Each area should be blocked off and signs should identify the purpose of each area.

Recommended components of PPE:

- PAPR- Powered Air Purifying Respirator- this type of respirator uses a battery-operated blower to pass contaminated air through a HEPA filter which removes the contaminant and supplies purified air to a face piece.
- Disposable N-95 or N-100 respirator can be used instead of a PAPR.
- Disposable single-use hood that extends to the shoulders and completely covers the neck.
- Disposable single-use fluid-resistant gown that extends to at least mid-calf.

- Disposable coverall with or without integrated socks can be used instead of the gown.
- Disposable nitrile examination gloves with extended cuffs- 2 pairs should be worn.
- Disposable fluid-resistant boot covers or shoe covers that extend to at least mid-calf.
- Disposable fluid-resistant apron that covers from the torso to mid-calf should be used in Ebola patients with bleeding, vomiting, or diarrhea.

Procedure for putting on PPE:

- Have a trained observer who will visually confirm that all equipment is serviceable and has been put on correctly. A written checklist will be used to confirm compliance with each step of the protocol. No exposed skin or visible hair should be seen when all PPE has been put on correctly.
- Remove all personal clothing and items. Change into surgical scrubs or disposable garments. No jewelry or personal items should be worn in the patient's room. Cell phones, beepers, pens, flashlights, and scissors should not be brought into the patient's room.
- Visually inspect each item of PPE to ensure it is serviceable and that all components are available prior to donning them.
- Perform hand hygiene with an alcohol-based hand sanitizer. Make sure your hands are clean and completely dry before moving to the next step.
- Put on your inner gloves.
- Put on your boots or shoe covers.
- Put on your gown or coverall. Make sure it is large enough for unrestricted movement. Make sure your inner gloves are tucked under the sleeve of the gown or coverall.
- Put on your outer gloves with extended cuffs. Make sure they are pulled over the sleeves of the gown or coverall.
- Put on your respirator.

- Put on your disposable hood and make sure it extends to the shoulders and fully covers your neck.
- Put on your full-length disposable apron if you are at risk of exposure to the patient's body fluids.
- Verify that all the equipment is serviceable and that all skin and hair is covered. Make sure you can extend your arms, bend at the waist, and move freely. Make sure that all of the PPE remains in place while you are moving.
- Disinfect your outer gloves and let them dry thoroughly prior to patient contact.

Once all items of PPE has been carefully put on and both the healthcare worker and trained observer have completed the checklist and visually inspected the PPE for integrity and intactness- the healthcare worker can enter the patient's room. All necessary care will be performed by the healthcare worker. He will be careful to avoid exposure or contamination while care is given. Once care for the Ebola patient is completed- the health care worker will proceed to the designated area for removing PPE. If there is any accidental breach in PPE procedure- the healthcare worker will go immediately to the area where PPE is removed to assess the exposure and implement the facility exposure plan.

Procedure for taking off PPE:

- Removing PPE should be done under the supervision of a trained observer as he reads aloud each step of the procedure and confirms visually that each item has been removed properly and according to the protocol. The trained observer should remind the health care worker to avoid reflexive actions that could cause exposure like touching the face or scratching the skin.
- Inspect the PPE for correct placement of each piece and look for any cuts or tears in the equipment. If any PPE is visibly contaminated- disinfect use an EPA-approved disinfectant wipe.
- Disinfect the outer gloves with an EPA-approved disinfectant wipe or alcohol-based hand sanitizer.
- Remove and **discard the apron** if it was used. Roll the apron from inside to outside to avoid contaminating the gloves.

- Inspect the remaining items of PPE for cuts, tears, or visible contamination. Disinfect any visibly contaminated item of PPE using an EPA-approved disinfectant wipe.
- Disinfect the outer gloves with an EPA-approved disinfectant wipe or alcohol-based hand sanitizer.
- Sit down to **remove the boots or shoe covers**.
- Disinfect the outer gloves with an EPA-approved disinfectant wipe or alcohol-based hand sanitizer. **Remove and discard the outer gloves** taking care not to contaminate the inner gloves during the removal process.
- Inspect the inner gloves' outer surfaces for cuts, tears, or visible contamination. If an inner glove is visibly soiled, cut, or torn- disinfect the inner gloves with an EPA-approved disinfectant wipe or alcohol-based hand sanitizer. Don a clean pair of gloves for the rest of the procedure. If there was no soiling, cuts, or tears on visual inspection of the inner gloves- disinfect the inner gloves with an EPA-approved disinfectant wipe or alcohol-based hand sanitizer.
- **Remove the face shield**. Avoid touching it's front surface.
- Disinfect the inner gloves with an EPA-approved disinfectant wipe or alcohol-based hand sanitizer.
- **Remove the surgical hood**.
- Disinfect the inner gloves with an EPA-approved disinfectant wipe or alcohol-based hand sanitizer.
- **Remove the gown or coverall.** Avoid contact with your scrubs or disposable garments as you remove the gown or coverall. Roll the garment from the inside out while touching only the inside of the gown or coverall.
- Disinfect the inner gloves with an EPA-approved disinfectant wipe or alcohol-based hand sanitizer. Remove and discard your gloves taking care not to contaminate your bare hands during the removal process. Perform hand hygiene with an alcohol-based hand sanitizer. Put on a new pair of inner gloves.
- **Remove the N95 respirator**.

- Disinfect the inner gloves with an EPA-approved disinfectant wipe or alcohol-based hand sanitizer.
- Disinfect washable shoes. Sitting on a clean surface use an EPA-approved disinfectant wipe to wipe down every external surface of the washable shoes.
- **Disinfect and remove inner gloves.** Disinfect the inner gloves with an EPA-approved disinfectant wipe or alcohol-based hand sanitizer. Remove and discard the gloves taking care not to contaminate the bare hands while removing the gloves.
- Perform hand hygiene with alcohol-based hand sanitizer.
- Perform a final visual inspection of the healthcare worker to look for signs of contamination of the surgical scrubs or disposable garments. If any signs of contamination are noted- the infection prevention specialist or the OSHA coordinator must be notified before exiting the PPE removal area.
- If all procedures for removal of PPE were followed correctly and documented according to the protocol and no signs of contamination are present- the healthcare worker can leave the PPE area wearing dedicated washable footwear and surgical scrubs or disposable garments.

Review of procedure and end of shift requirements:

- Either the infection prevention specialist, the OSHA coordinator or a designee should meet with the healthcare worker to review the patient care activities performed and identify any concerns about the care protocols. Evaluation of the fatigue and stress status of the healthcare worker should also be evaluated.
- Showers are recommended at the end of the shift for any healthcare worker who performs high risk patient care- especially if exposure to blood or body fluids is likely. Staff who spend extended periods of time in the room of an Ebola patient for any reason are encouraged to shower before leaving the unit.

Healthcare workers who are working with infectious Ebola patients are giving high risk care and working in a stressful environment. They are heroes who are risking Ebola exposure and infection. Show them your appreciation with a pat on the back and thank them for their courage and leadership.

Chapter 18
Recommendations for Travelers to Western Africa

Ebola disease is pandemic in regions of West Africa. The CDC has issued a Level 3 travel notice- advising people to avoid non-essential travel to Guinea, Sierra Leone, Liberia, and Mali. This means that there is significant risk of exposure to Ebola virus when travelers visit these countries. The safest practice is to avoid travel to any areas of West Africa that have outbreaks of Ebola disease. When travel to West Africa cannot be avoided- these are CDC recommendations which will protect you from exposure to Ebola virus:

- Make sure your vaccinations up-to-date.
- Be sure you are healthy and free of infectious disease.
- Take your usual vitamins and medications.
- Wash your hands frequently with soap and water.
- Alcohol-based hand sanitizer may be used if soap and water is not available for hand-washing.
- Cover open wounds or sores.
- Do not touch bats, non-human primates, or any bush animals.
- Avoid animal blood or body secretions.
- Do not handle or consume raw or cooked bush meat.
- Do not go into remote villages of the bush or on safari.
- Wear a facemask, goggles, and gloves if you have contact with someone who is sick.
- Avoid villages where Ebola disease has been diagnosed.
- Avoid medical facilities where Ebola patients are being cared for.
- Avoid contact with the blood or body secretions of anyone- especially those who are ill.
- Do not handle items that have been contaminated with body secretions from someone known to have Ebola disease such as clothing, bedding, needles, or contaminated medical equipment used during their treatment.

- Do not touch the body of anyone who has died from Ebola disease or any suspicious cause.
- Avoid sexual contact with unknown or native partners.
- If you are on a humanitarian aid mission to Western Africa- follow all the instructions of your humanitarian aid organization, the CDC, and the public health authorities.
- Seek medical care immediately if you develop fever, headache, muscle pain, joint pain, fatigue, vomiting, diarrhea, stomach pain, or unexplained bruising or bleeding.
- Go immediately to a hospital if you have symptoms of Ebola disease and you had exposure to someone who was diagnosed with Ebola disease.
- IF you were exposed to someone with Ebola disease- limit your contact with other people until you have been medically evaluated and released from care.
- Submit gracefully to the enhanced screening and monitoring measures that are being taken at the airports and entry points to the United States and other countries. Their goal is to prevent Ebola virus transmission to other countries around the world.
- Follow all guidelines and recommendations of the CDC and the WHO.

Chapter 19

Screening Travelers Returning to the United States

The CDC, Department of Homeland Security, Department of Transportation, and Customs and Border Patrol are taking active measures to prevent ill travelers from entering the United States. Protecting US citizens from Ebola virus exposure and preventing Ebola disease are the top health priorities in the United States.

The CDC has been working with airlines, airports, and ministries of health in all West African countries with widespread Ebola disease to detect travelers who are sick or who have been exposed to Ebola virus. The goal is to prevent them from boarding a commercial flight until it is safe for them to travel.

Exit screening protocols: may look a little different in different countries but these are the basic elements of exit screening. Any traveler who is leaving Guinea, Liberia, Sierra Leone, or Mali and anyone who had a stop in any of these countries while travelling will have exit screening prior to departure from Western Africa.

These travelers will:

- Have their temperatures taken.
- Answer questions about their health and exposure history.
- Be visually assessed for signs of illness.

Travelers with possible exposure or symptoms will be separated and assessed further. The results of this assessment will determine whether they are allowed to travel or detained for an incubation period of up to 21 days past their last exposure. Anyone who has been exposed to Ebola within the last 21 days will not be allowed to fly on a commercial flight. Anyone with symptoms of Ebola disease must be referred to public health authorities for further evaluation.

United States Department of Transportation rules permit airlines to deny boarding to air travelers with serious contagious diseases that could worsen or spread during the flight- including travelers with symptoms of Ebola disease. This rule applies to all flights of US airlines and to direct flights to or from the United States by foreign airlines.

Travelers who become ill while traveling: will be asked by airline crews if they were in Guinea, Liberia, Sierra Leone, or Mali in the last 21 days. If the traveler denies travel or stopovers in these countries and has no other risk factors that indicate increased exposure risk- routine infection control precautions will be used in his care during the flight. Any traveler that has had exposure and has symptoms suggestive of Ebola disease must be reported immediately to the CDC.

Certain measures should be taken during the flight for any ill passenger including:

- Keeping sick travelers separated from other passengers as much as possible.
- Wear waterproof disposable gloves before directly touching him or cleaning blood or body fluids.
- Do not give a surgical mask to anyone who is nauseated or vomiting.
- Encourage ill passengers who are not nauseated or vomiting to wear a surgical mask.
- Give an air sickness bag to anyone who is nauseated or vomiting.
- Encourage anyone who is coughing and sneezing to cover their mouth and nose.
- Use a plastic bag for disposal of used tissues or air sick bags.
- Cabin crew should follow infection control principles and use full PPE from the Universal Precautions Kit if a passenger is ill and has traveled through any country with widespread Ebola disease or if he has had Ebola virus exposure and is symptomatic.

- Hand hygiene should be used frequently while caring for an ill passenger.
- All body fluids should be treated as if they were infectious.
- Pilots of international flights inbound to the United are required by law to report any on-board deaths or ill travelers with certain symptoms to the CDC.

The risk to passengers or crew members of getting Ebola disease from an ill traveler is very low because Ebola is not an airborne disease. Direct contact with the blood or body fluids from a person with symptomatic Ebola disease is required to transmit Ebola virus. If a traveler has confirmed Ebola disease and was on a commercial flight to the United States- the CDC will conduct an investigation to assess risk and alert the passengers and airline crew of possible exposure.

Entry screening in the United States: The CDC is working closely with Customs at US Airports and Border Patrol units at border crossings into the United States to screen people who have symptoms of contagious diseases-including Ebola.

The Department of Homeland Security (DHS) and the Center for Disease Control (CDC) have designated five major airport hubs in the United States as entry points for flights originating from Western Africa. These airports are JFK Airport in New York, Newark Airport in New Jersey, Dulles Airport in Washington DC, O'Hare Airport in Chicago, and Hartsville-Jackson Airport in Atlanta. Using these major hubs as entry points for high risk flights and using enhanced screening techniques are predicted to successfully screen over 94% of commercial airline travelers returning from countries infected with widespread Ebola disease.

These are the basic components of the CDC's enhanced screening protocol for travelers returning from Guinea, Liberia, Sierra Leone, Mali, or any passengers suspected of having potentially infectious diseases:

- Each passenger at risk will receive a CARE kit that includes a thermometer, symptom card, and log book to enter the results of the daily health checks for 21 days past the last potential exposure to Ebola virus.

- Temperature will be taken twice a day- in the morning and evening.
- Daily symptom checks will look for fever, headache, muscle or joint pain, increased fatigue or weakness, vomiting, diarrhea, stomach pain, or unusual bruising or bleeding.
- A public health worker will come to your home for direct assessment of your condition once a day if you are considered at high risk and in need of direct active monitoring by the public health department.
- A public healthcare worker will contact you once or twice a day for active monitoring if your assessed level of risk requires public health assessment. They will review your temperature, symptoms, and general health.

If you think you have had Ebola exposure and you have symptoms suggestive of Ebola disease:

- You must follow the recommendations of the public health care worker who contacts you.
- Do not be afraid. Seek medical care to protect yourself, your family, and your community.
- If you have had Ebola virus exposure and become very sick- call 911 and the hospital. Warn them about the Ebola exposure so they are ready to take appropriate infection control precautions and so they can plan for appropriate triage and care in the Emergency Room.
- Do not take public transportation.
- Do not go to social outings.
- Do not go to work, church, or school.

Chapter 20
Health Care in West African Villages

Managing Ebola disease in the villages and bush of Western Africa is complicated and dangerous but it is absolutely critical. Africa is ground zero for Ebola virus. Ebola is pandemic in Western Africa- but there have been very few cases outside of Africa's borders. Keeping Ebola virus contained in Western Africa and preventing transmission to other continents and countries will determine the fate of the world.

All nations, governments, and humanitarian aid organizations have joined hands in co-operation to help Western Africa fight against Ebola. Relief efforts during the 2014 West African pandemic have been more extensive than for any other infectious disease outbreak in history.

The CDC has set a timeline of January 1, 2015 to have measures in place that will contain the Ebola pandemic that is raging in Western Africa. The plan calls for:

- Isolation of 100% of Ebola infected patients.
- Isolate all contacts and quarantine villages and communities with exposure risk for a 21 day isolation period from their last known exposure.
- Build Ebola Treatment Centers (ETCs) that are specialized and fully stocked with personnel and supplies to manage patients with Ebola disease in cities.
- Build Community Care Center (CCCs) in remote villages of the bush to isolate all Ebola cases in small localized geographical areas. CCCs are smaller and more mobile than ETCs. They

generally have 8-15 beds per facility and are able to provide safe care for African villagers by trained personnel.

- Consistent practice of strong infection control procedures that are practiced correctly by personnel who are fully trained and 100% compliant.
- Provide safe burials for 100% of the patients who die of Ebola disease.

The CDC and WHO have established guidelines for managing care in remote villages of the bush. Field hospitals and CCCs are being set up to triage and treat patients with Ebola disease. All healthcare facilities performing triage and care for patients with Ebola exposure or disease must have the following specific areas:

- Screening area- screening should take place outside but near the entrance to the clinic or healthcare facility. All entry into the clinic or hospital should be through this entrance and all other entry points should be blocked off and inaccessible. Set up a wooden table and two wooden chairs at least 5 feet apart. Set up supplies needed to screen patients such as a hand hygiene station with weakly chlorinated water, soap, alcohol-based hand sanitizer, a hand-washing poster, two or more working thermometers, disposable towels, disposable nitrile gloves, full face shields or face masks and goggles, a screening flowchart, and a small waste bin for disposable used waste. All patients must perform hand hygiene on arrival at the screening site following the guidelines on the hand-washing poster.
- Clean area (considered a cold area)–for non-suspected patients and staff- traditional care will be performed there with several exceptions. Hand-washing stations will be set up throughout the clean area and hand hygiene will be encouraged. Basic PPE will be available and used when caring for any patient. This includes boots, gloves, goggles, and face mask.
- Isolation area (considered a hot area)–this area should be separated from the regular clinic and will only be used for suspected Ebola cases. It cannot be used for routine treatment of non-suspect patients or storage of supplies or equipment. The

isolation room should be separated from all other areas of the building or it can be a separate tent that is set up outside at a distance from the healthcare facility. It should be marked with signs for patients and staff to know that it is an isolation area and only authorized personnel are allowed to enter. A guard should be placed near the entrance/exit to prevent unauthorized entry into this area. A log book should be used to identify healthcare workers who enter the area and what task or procedure they performed. There should be simple beds and non-upholstered furniture to allow easy and effective disinfection. Mattresses must be protected with plastic covers. Any furnishings, bedding, or clothing provided by the family must be burned after the patient leaves unless it can be disinfected. Buckets with strong and weak chlorine for disinfection and cleaning should be available in the isolation area. Feeding utensils should be clearly marked for use in the isolation area and each patient should have his own utensils. A latrine or commode bucket should be clearly marked for use by suspected Ebola patients only. A bedpan may be substituted when no latrine or commode is available. Only personnel trained and designated to work in the isolation area should be allowed to enter the area and the number of times the isolation area is entered should be minimized. Full PPE is used at all times in the isolation area.

- An area to put on PPE- This area should be clearly identified and only used to put on PPE. It should be outside the isolation area and have adequate supplies available. There should be a poster showing how to put on PPE correctly. There should be a hand washing station with mild chlorine solution for disinfection and hand hygiene. PPE should be available including gowns, disposable gloves, face shields or goggles and face mask, gloves, head covering, aprons, and thick reusable gloves.
- An area to take off PPE- this area should be clearly identified and only used to take off PPE. It should be outside the isolation area and have adequate supplies available. There should be a poster showing how to take off PPE correctly. A bucket filled with strong chlorine solution should be available to soak goggles, aprons, and dirty reusable gloves. A glove-washing station should be set up

with a strong chlorine solution. Weak chlorine solution should be used for rinsing reusable PPE items after they have soaked. A foot bath should be filled with strong chlorine solution to wash boots. There should be a container with a lid to hold infectious waste that will be incinerated. PPE removal should be supervised by someone trained in using PPE correctly. They will watch for potential breaches in the protocol. There should be a hand hygiene station for hand-washing after PPE has been completely removed. Disposable towels should be available for use.

- Areas for toilets or latrines- Latrines for non-suspect patients and staff must be kept separate from latrines used by suspected or confirmed Ebola patients. Signs should clearly indicate who can use each area where toilets or latrines are located.
- Waste management area- there should be an area of the clinic or hospital grounds marked off for waste management. This area should not be in a high flow area or in areas that attract attention. All disposable waste of any healthcare facility will be burned in a burn pit or incinerator.

It is important to have a consistent layout and design for clinics and hospitals where Ebola patients are cared for. Separating clean areas from potentially infectious areas helps minimize the risk of contamination and exposure to Ebola virus. Health care workers can perform their duties knowing that all staff members are complying with infection control guidelines correctly and consistently.

Chapter 21
Health Care for Ebola Patients in US Hospitals

The Ebola pandemic in Western Africa continues to rage. Cases of Ebola disease are continuing to grow rapidly. Mortality rates in Western Africa remain consistent at about 60%. The world continues to look at the Ebola crisis in Africa and asks: Is my country next? Is my family safe here? Do the government, the health authorities, and the medical community have my back? What if...

The risk of Ebola disease in the United States is very low. Only health care workers who have cared for patients with symptomatic Ebola disease have been infected while they were in the United States. Our health care system is one of the most advanced and sophisticated in the world. We have up-to-date technology, unsurpassed diagnostic capabilities, and skilled and well-trained health care workers.

Our government, the national public health system, our medical community, and the CDC are vigilant and ready to care for anyone in the United States who has been exposed to Ebola virus or has Ebola disease. Procedures and protocols have been established to ensure safe care for every patient with Ebola disease in the United States. Many of the CDC's guidelines and recommendations have already been discussed and should be reviewed from previous chapters.

These are **general guidelines** for managing people who are ill in any health care setting:

- Identify anyone with Ebola virus exposure.
- Isolate anyone with Ebola virus exposure who is not symptomatic for a 21 day incubation period from their last exposure.
- Contacts of anyone with symptomatic Ebola disease must be investigated by the public health department.
- Quarantine and 21 day monitoring and movement protocols need to be enforced for all contacts of patients with confirmed Ebola disease.

- Anyone with known Ebola virus exposure who is having symptoms of Ebola disease should be hospitalized for evaluation and medical treatment.
- All confirmed cases of Ebola disease must be reported to the hospital's infectious diseases department, the local and state public health department, and the CDC.
- Medical care must be provided in an environment that is safe for the patient and the health care workers.
- Infection control measures should include isolation, hand hygiene, and consistent and correct use of personal protective equipment by all people having contact with suspected or confirmed Ebola patients.
- Care should be taken when handling sharp objects like used needles and scalpels.
- Disposable medical equipment and supplies that are contaminated should be incinerated.
- Re-usable equipment and medical supplies should be cleaned and disinfected according to the manufacturer's instructions and the hospital's policy.
- Cleaning and disinfecting the patient's environment should be done with disinfectants suitable for use with Ebola virus and the product should be used according to the label's instructions.
- The facility should be compliant with all relevant policies and procedures of the local and state public health department, the CDC, OSHA, and the EPA.

Ebola Treatment Centers (ETCs):

Thirty five hospitals in the United States have been designated as Ebola treatment centers (ETCs). These hospitals will provide state-of-the-art comprehensive care for Ebola patients from admission to discharge. Each center has passed a comprehensive site visit by the CDC and has shown competency, proficiency, and expertise in all service areas required to care for Ebola patients.

ETCs must have readiness plans that are established by a multi-disciplinary team including members from every department involved in caring for

Ebola patients. These are some of the capabilities required for a facility to be designated as an ETC:

- ETC's must be staffed with healthcare workers from all departments of the hospital on a 24/7 basis. The Ebola care team includes health care providers giving direct patient care at the bedside such as physicians, infection control specialists, pharmacists, critical care nurses, nursing assistants, respiratory therapists, laboratory technicians, EMS, and pathologists. The team also includes members who do not give direct face-to-face care but assist in ancillary roles such as dietary, environmental services, laundry, security, maintenance, clerical workers, chaplains, and volunteers. Even the behind-the- scenes personnel who do not have direct contact with patients can be exposed to infectious agents through contact with health care workers or contaminated medical equipment. Every health care worker assigned to the Ebola care team is there voluntarily, has been fully trained, and has demonstrated competency to perform their job safely.
- ETCs must have ongoing training and quality assurance programs to monitor compliance with infection control measures, safe and correct PPE usage, proper waste management, appropriate decontamination and disinfection procedures, and proper collection and handling of laboratory specimens.
- ETC's have a designated site manager in the location where the Ebola patient is cared for. He is on-site in the Ebola unit at all times. His sole responsibility is to provide safe and effective treatment for the Ebola patient and ensure the safety of health care personnel.
- ETCs have worker safety policies and programs that are in compliance with all federal and state occupational safety and health (OSHA) standards. ECUs have a procedure that ensures direct active monitoring of all health care workers involved in Ebola patient care for 21 days past their last exposure. The monitoring will be done in coordination with the local and state public health agencies.

- ETC's must have a trained observer who supervises putting on and taking off PPE **every time** patient care is given using a designated procedure checklist. The facility must have sufficient stores of PPE to last at least seven days.
- ETCs have a facility plan and an agreed on method for communicating with local and state public health authorities and the CDC. All patients under investigation (PUI) for Ebola disease and all patients with a confirmed diagnosis of Ebola disease have been reported to the local and state public health authorities and the CDC. Both organizations are involved in case management on a consultation basis.
- ETCs must have laboratory procedures and protocols that provide for safe specimen collection and transport. The lab must be capable of performing all diagnostic tests to confirm Ebola disease and any specialized tests required to assess the medical condition of an Ebola patient.
- ETC's must have intra-facility transfer plans coordinated with state and local public health agencies and EMS providers. The EMS provider must have personnel with infection control expertise and PPE must always be used. EMS will transfer Ebola patients when needed to ensure exceptional health care at specialized facilities.
- ETC's must have a program in place to clean and disinfect patient care areas and equipment using Environmental Protection Agency (EPA) approved disinfectants. The staff must be trained in safe cleaning of the patient care environment and correct use of PPE. Environmental services staff are always under direct supervision while performing cleaning and disinfection in the patient care environment.
- ETC's must use waste management services capable of managing and transporting Category A infectious substances and must have appropriate containers and procedures for safe temporary storage of Category A waste. The staff must be trained in safe PPE use and proper handling and storage techniques.

Ebola Triage Protocol:

Outpatient ambulatory care settings such as clinics, physician's offices, ambulance services, and emergency rooms may need to evaluate patients who have symptoms consistent with early Ebola disease. Any patient who presents with flu-like symptoms and has exam findings consistent with viral illness should have a travel and exposure history taken.

Travel History: Has the patient lived in or traveled to a country with widespread Ebola disease in the last 21 days?

Exposure History: Has the patient had contact with someone who has confirmed Ebola disease? Has he been exposed to Ebola virus in the last 21 days?

A patient who does not give a suspicious travel or exposure history should have routine triage assessment and testing. Anyone who has traveled in areas of West Africa with widespread Ebola disease or had exposure to Ebola virus or a patient with symptomatic Ebola disease needs to be aggressively triaged to make sure he does not have early Ebola disease.

Identify signs and symptoms of early Ebola disease. Does the patient have fever > 100.5 degrees, fatigue, headache, weakness, muscle pain, vomiting, diarrhea, abdominal pain, bruising, or bleeding? If no signs of Ebola disease are noted- continue with routine triage assessment but notify the public health department about his triage visit so he can be monitored for fever and symptoms for 21 days.

Any person with a positive travel history or known exposure to Ebola- becomes a **person under investigation (PUI).** These patients are suspicious for Ebola disease and need to be screened thoroughly to determine the cause of their illness.

- Isolate the patient in a private room with a private bathroom.
- Activate the hospital preparedness plan for Ebola.
- Do diagnostic testing for Ebola disease.
- Consider and screen the patient for alternative causes of his infection.
- Notify the infectious diseases department of the hospital.
- Notify the public health department.

- Use strict infection control procedures to minimize the risk of Ebola virus exposure.
- Only essential personnel should have contact with the patient.
- PPE should be used for every patient care encounter.
- Family members and visitors must wear PPE.
- Use disposable and dedicated equipment that is not shared with other patients.
- Create a clinical care team led by a senior level experienced clinician that includes a hospital infection control specialist, an infectious disease specialist, a senior nurse, and a senior critical care specialist.
- Assign a senior staff member of the clinical care team to coordinate test results from the hospital lab, the state public health department lab, and the CDC. He should coordinate all communication and reporting between the ETC and local and state health organizations.
- When the outpatient setting is not a hospital capable of managing the care of an Ebola patient- arrangements must be made to transfer the patient to the nearest hospital or ETC capable of caring for him. Every organization involved in the transfer must know that the patient is under investigation for Ebola disease so that appropriate precautions can be taken. All state and local authorities must be notified of an Ebola patient's transfer including law enforcement and public health authorities at the transferring and receiving facilities.

Any patients whose laboratory testing comes back positive for Ebola disease becomes a **confirmed Ebola case**. Reporting confirmed cases of Ebola disease to all public health agencies and the CDC is mandatory. It begins the process of providing medical care for the Ebola patient, identifying and isolating his contacts, and investigating the need for quarantine or monitoring and movement restrictions.

The United States has well established and effective Ebola policies and procedures that are designed to ensure the health and well-being of every US citizen. Safe and effective care of Ebola patients in the United States is a top health priority. Any patient with Ebola disease will get excellent medical care in a well-staffed and up-to-date medical facility. He and his family will receive compassionate care and they will be treated with dignity and respect. He will get the medical expertise and help he needs to become an Ebola survivor.

Chapter 22
Safe Burials in Western Africa

The World Health Organization (WHO) has developed a protocol to ensure safe burials of patients who died from suspected or confirmed Ebola disease. Burial traditions are very important to families and communities who lose a loved one. Burials have cultural and religious significance and are deeply personal and meaningful. When people are not allowed to grieve in their usual manner and say goodbye in their own personal way- conflict can erupt and escalate into violent confrontations between villagers and aid workers who are there to bury the dead.

Burial teams have been assembled in Western Africa to ensure safe burials that are culturally sensitive. The goal is to honor the dead and show respect to his family, community, and culture while ensuring a safe burial of his potentially infectious body. Only trained members of the burial team should have contact with human remains and touching and handling the body should be kept to a minimum.

Guidelines to follow when conducting a **culturally sensitive burial:**

- The team leader should brief the burial team about the religious and cultural beliefs of the community where the deceased lived.
- The burial team should not wear PPE on arrival.
- Burial teams should include a sprayer, a technical supervisor, a communicator, and a religious representative.
- The team should greet the family and offer condolences before unloading necessary equipment and supplies.
- Respectfully request a family representative.
- Contact the local faith representative at the family's request to meet the burial team at the place of collection of the deceased. If the community has no faith leader- the team supervisor can contact someone from a list of faith representatives at the family's request.
- The communicator and the faith representative will work together with the family representative to make sure that the burial is

carried out in a culturally sensitive manner that honors the deceased, his family, and his community.

- The burial team will wait until all communication has concluded, all questions have been answered, and the family has formally agreed to the burial.
- Identify family members who will participate in burial rituals such as prayers, orations, dancing, chanting, wailing, or closing the coffin.
- If the family has chosen a coffin- identify four family members who will carry it.
- Make sure the grave has been dug. Send someone to dig it at the cemetery or place chosen by the family if needed.
- Invite one or two family members to witness the preparation of the body for burial.
- Ask if there are specific requests from the family or community about the personal effects of the deceased (burn, bury in the grave, or disinfect).
- Accept any rituals that are consistent with the faith and beliefs of the family unless they require contact with the body.
- Allow the family to take pictures of the preparation and burial. Offer the services of a member of the burial team to take pictures on their behalf if the family desires.
- Ask the family if they have an item to identify the grave like an identity plaque, headstone, cross, or photograph of the deceased.

Guidelines to follow when conducting a **safe burial**:

- Assemble all equipment and supplies that are needed before entering the room where the body is located.
- Infection control measures and PPE should be used correctly and consistently during all burials.
- Open all windows and doors for optimal light and ventilation.
- Evaluate the size and weight of the deceased to choose the right size body bag. Body bags should be opaque.
- Place the coffin outside the house if chosen by the family.

- Identify all areas of the house and any outside structures such as community bathrooms or toilets that were used by the deceased patient so they can be cleaned and disinfected.
- Put on all personal protective equipment used by the burial team in the presence of the family.
- Enter the house respectfully.
- Collect post mortem epidemiological samples for confirmation of Ebola disease.
- Place the body bag beside the deceased and open it.
- Two people will place deceased in the body bag using the arms and legs then close the body bag.
- Outer surfaces of the body bag will be disinfected with a sprayer containing a suitable disinfectant.
- **Human remains should never be sprayed, washed, or embalmed. Manipulation of the body must be minimal.**
- Transport the body bag to the coffin.
- Place the burial clothing and objects that are to be buried with the deceased in the coffin if the family desires.
- Allow one of the family members to close the coffin lid wearing gloves.
- Respect the grief of the family and give them time to say good-bye.
- Disinfect the coffin.
- When there is no burial planned- place the body bag in the rear of the pickup vehicle with the head toward the front.
- Collect sharp objects that might have been used on the deceased and dispose of them in a leak-proof and puncture resistant container.
- Clean and disinfect all rooms of the house and annex that were used by the deceased. Special attention should be given to areas soiled with blood and body secretions.

- Clean and disinfect all objects that may have been touched by the deceased.
- Gather bed linen, clothes, and possessions of the deceased that need to be discarded. Place them in a plastic bag that is tightly closed and disinfect the outside of the bag.
- Mattresses, mats, soiled linens, and clothing used by the deceased must be burned a safe distance from the house. Make sure the family has agreed to the incineration. **The burial team will give the family new mattresses and mats**.
- Review to make sure that all areas of the house and any areas of the community that the deceased used have been cleaned and disinfected and that all contaminated articles have been removed from the home.
- Remove PPE.
- Perform hand hygiene.
- Communicate your condolences to the family and answer any questions they have.
- Household gloves will be used to carry the disinfected coffin to the transport vehicle or the cemetery if it is nearby. Distribute gloves to family members who have been designated to carry the coffin. Place the coffin delicately in the transport vehicle with the head toward the front of the vehicle.
- Respect the grief of the family and allow them adequate time to sing, chant, pray, wail, and remember their loved one.
- Allow family members to sit in the rear of the transport vehicle with the deceased but only the burial team may sit in the closed cab of the vehicle.
- Any other participants will follow the vehicle carrying the deceased on foot.
- The funeral processional should be handled according to the traditions of the community.
- Manually carry the coffin to the gravesite that has been chosen by the family.

- Lower the coffin or body bag into the grave.
- Place the belongings of the deceased that were chosen by the family into the grave.
- Allow the family to say goodbye in their unique way and respect their mourning rituals.
- Allow family members to close the grave if that is their preference.
- Place identification on the grave and a religious symbol if the family requests.
- Recover all household gloves that were used by the family or burial team.
- The burial team should attend the funeral, offer condolences to the family, and may offer small gifts of respect to honor the deceased family member.
- The family, community members, and burial team should have a communal hand washing with soap and water or alcohol based sanitizer. Each person who attended the funeral should participate.
- The burial team should offer their final condolences and answer any questions of the family.
- All equipment and supplies will be assembled and stored.
- The burial team will leave the premises respectfully.

Chapter 23

Managing Human Remains in the United States

These are the CDC's recommendations for handling human remains of people with suspected or confirmed Ebola disease in hospital morgues and commercial mortuaries in the United States. When anyone dies of Ebola disease- their body is capable of transmitting Ebola virus to healthy people who provide postmortem care. The greatest risk of infection comes from handling human remains without personal protective equipment (PPE), splashes of infected blood or body fluids, and lacerations or puncture with contaminated instruments during postmortem procedures.

General guidelines:

- Only personnel who are trained in handling infected human remains and are wearing PPE should touch or move Ebola infected remains.
- Handling of human remains should be kept to a minimum.
- Autopsies on patients who die of Ebola disease should be avoided when the diagnosis was confirmed. When autopsy is deemed to be necessary- the public health department and the CDC should be consulted regarding whether additional precautions should be taken.

Postmortem care personnel:

- Should wear PPE for the duration of any procedure that requires contact with human remains.
- Should use caution when removing PPE to avoid accidental contamination of the wearer.

- Should perform hand hygiene immediately after removing PPE with soap and water if hands or visibly soiled or with an alcohol-based hand sanitizer if there is no obvious soiling of the hands.

Postmortem preparation:

- The body should be wrapped in a plastic shroud in a way that prevents contamination of the outside of the shroud.
- Gowns and gloves should be changed if they become heavily contaminated with blood or body fluids.
- Leave intravenous lines or endotracheal tubes in place if they are present.
- Avoid washing or cleaning the body.
- Place the body in a leak-proof body bag and make sure it is zippered closed. A leak-proof bag is puncture-resistant and sealed in a way that prevents leakage of contents during handling, transport, and shipping of the body.
- Place the body in a second leak-proof body bag and make sure it is zippered completely shut.
- Disinfect and decontaminate the outside of the corpse-containing body bag according to the instructions on the disinfectant's label and allow to air dry.
- Transport the body to the morgue.
- The patient room should be cleaned and disinfected according to CDC recommended guidelines and hospital policy.
- Re-usable equipment should be cleaned and disinfected according to the manufacturer's instructions and the hospital policy.
- Personnel that are driving or riding in transport vehicles carrying human remains do not need to wear PPE if they will not be handling the body and if the remains have been handled using the procedure outlined above.

Mortuary Care:

- Bodies infected with Ebola disease should not be embalmed.
- Do not open the body bags.

- Do not remove remains from the body bag.
- Bagged bodies should be placed directly into a hermetically sealed casket (one that is airtight and does not allow escape of infectious microorganisms). The casket should have valid documentation that it is hermetically sealed and the seal should be intact on inspection.
- Wear full PPE including surgical scrub suit, surgical cap, impervious gown with full sleeves, eye protection, facemask, shoe covers, and double gloves when handling the bagged human remains.
- If leakage of body fluids occurs- thoroughly clean and decontaminate all area of the environment with EPA-registered disinfectants capable of killing Ebola virus according to the product's label instructions.

Disposition of human remains:

- Human remains should be cremated or buried promptly in a hermetically sealed casket.
- When a body bag containing human remains has been placed in a hermetically sealed casket- no additional cleaning or precautions need to be taken unless the seal is broken or leakage of body fluids has occurred.
- PPE is not needed when handling cremated remains or a hermetically sealed casket.

Transporting human remains:

- Transportation of Ebola infected remains should be minimized.
- Transportation (including to the mortuary or for the burial) should be coordinated with relevant local and state authorities.
- Interstate travel should be coordinated with the CDC by calling the Emergency Operations Center.
- Mode of transportation (ground transport or airline transport) must be carefully considered.
- Transportation of human remains of Ebola disease victims outside the United States needs to comply with the regulations of the

destination country and should be coordinated in advance with relevant authorities.

Private closed-casket funeral services and personal family memorial services are common when someone dies of Ebola disease. Traditional funerals with viewings of the deceased and open casket services are not possible. Special care needs to be taken to preserve the hermetic seals of the casket. Transportation of the body of an Ebola victim for burial requires special authorization and the processional is accompanied by law enforcement and local and state authorities.

Chapter 24
Recommendations for Humanitarian Aid Workers

Humanitarian aid organizations play a critical role in the 2014 West Africa Ebola pandemic. The key to controlling Ebola disease is stopping the transmission of Ebola at its source. Healthcare workers and management experts with specialized skills and experience are needed desperately to provide aid to African countries with Ebola.

Every aid worker should be affiliated with a recognized humanitarian aid organization. Incidents of unrest and civil violence against aid workers have been reported in West Africa. Your organization should have policies and procedures in place to protect your health and wellbeing while you are on mission. Your organization should be aware of unfolding events in West Africa and be ready to protect the health and safety of their workers.

These are the CDC's guidelines for a humanitarian aid worker from any country who want to take part in relief efforts in West Africa.

Training and preparation: You should have a thorough knowledge of Ebola disease and understand

- Potential sources of Ebola virus exposure.
- Preventive measures that reduce your risk of exposure to Ebola virus.
- How Ebola virus is transmitted to others.
- Signs and symptoms of Ebola disease.
- Infection control measures that reduce the risk of exposure.

- Consistent and correct use of PPE.
- Guidelines for isolation or quarantine of contacts.
- Guidelines for caring for patients with confirmed Ebola disease.
- Guidelines for safely moving suspected Ebola patients to Ebola treatment units in the community or hospital.
- Guidelines for clean-up and disinfection of contaminated objects and homes.
- Guidelines for safe burials of Ebola victims.

Preparation for departure to the field:

- You should have been seen by a travel medicine specialist 4-6 weeks before you leave on mission.
- Pre-deployment health screens should be done to assess your health and emotional fitness to perform in a high risk and stressful environment.
- Your vaccinations must be current and you should have adequate supplies of any medications you may need while on mission.
- You should have PPE- including facemasks, gloves, gowns, eye protection, and shoe covers. You should know when to use PPE and how to use it correctly.
- Check on the status of your visa status and register with the US Embassy in your destination country.
- Know about your medical insurance and what is covered if you become ill in a foreign country. Make sure that you are covered for Ebola disease and that aid workers in West Africa are not excluded from coverage.
- Identify where you can get health care while in West Africa.
- Make prior arrangements for medical evacuation if you have a serious medical illness or injury while you are on mission.
- You will not be allowed on commercial flights to return home if you were exposed to a symptomatic patient with confirmed Ebola disease or if you are diagnosed with Ebola disease.

- Make sure your medical coverage includes emergency air evacuation. Ask about the costs, coverage limits, deductibles, and co-pays if you need to use emergency air evacuation. More information on medical evacuation can be found at http://travel.state.gov/content/passports/english/go/health/evacuation.html
- Ask whether you will be returned to the United States or the nearest location where adequate medical care if offered if you are diagnosed with Ebola disease.
- Know the procedure for reporting exposure or illness to your humanitarian aid organization.
- Understand how to self-monitor for Ebola disease while in West Africa and on return to your home country.
- Check your humanitarian aid organization's procedures about whether they will help you return home if you have had known exposure to Ebola virus but do not have symptoms. You will not be able to fly by commercial airlines- will you have access to a private charter service or will you have to wait the full 21 day incubation period before you are allowed to return home?

Recommendations for preventing Ebola disease while providing aid in West Africa

- Wash your hands with soap and water or an alcohol-based hand sanitizer frequently according to CDC guidelines.
- Avoid contact with blood or body fluids (such as urine, vomit, saliva, feces, sweat, semen, vaginal secretions, or breast milk) of someone with Ebola disease.
- Do not handle any items that might have come in contact with an infected person's blood or body fluids.
- Avoid direct contact with the body of someone who died of Ebola disease.
- Do not participate in funeral or burial rituals unless that is your designated assignment.
- Avoid contact with animals such as bats or primates whether they are alive or dead.
- Do not eat or handle bush meat.

- Avoid hospitals where Ebola patients are treated unless you are a designated health care worker and that is your designated assignment.
- Report any incident of Ebola exposure immediately to your humanitarian organization using their reporting procedure.

Guidelines for aid workers who are exposed to Ebola virus- with or without symptoms

- Notify your humanitarian organization immediately. Follow their designated procedures for aid workers with Ebola exposure.
- Begin self-monitoring for symptoms of Ebola disease for 21 days after your last known exposure. Take your temperature twice a day in the morning and evening and watch for symptoms such as fever >101.5, severe headache, weakness, joint and muscle pain, vomiting, diarrhea, stomach pain, or unexplained bruising or bleeding.
- Seek medical care immediately if you develop symptoms of Ebola disease.

After you return home from your aid mission:

- Monitor your health for 21 days if you were in a country with widespread Ebola disease.
- Take your temperature twice a day.
- Watch for symptoms of Ebola disease.

Recommendations for an aid worker who develops symptoms of Ebola disease:

- Seek medical care immediately.
- Notify EMS or your emergency room about your recent travel and symptoms before you arrive at their facility so they can prepare for your arrival and have an isolation room and needed supplies available.
- Avoid public transportation.
- Limit contact with people.
- Do not travel anywhere except to the hospital.

If you are considering going to Western Africa on a humanitarian aid mission you should carefully consider the risks as well as the rewards of helping Ebola victims. There is a risk of Ebola virus exposure and infection with Ebola disease. You may need to receive health care in remote villages of the bush if you get sick while you are assigned there. There is a risk that you might have to stay in Africa for monitoring and movement for up to 21 days when your mission is finished. You might not be able to leave West Africa by commercial airlines if you have had Ebola exposure. Your insurance plan may not cover any costs of Ebola care and will not cover the full cost. If you contract Ebola disease you may need to be air-lifted out of Africa which may be very expensive if your aid organization does not pay for it.

Consider your decision carefully and use the guidelines given to determine your risks. Find out the facts and pre-plan for your mission before you leave. Carefully consider the implications of being infected with Ebola disease in Western Africa. Make sure your humanitarian agency has safety procedures and a contingency plan for transporting ill humanitarian workers home.

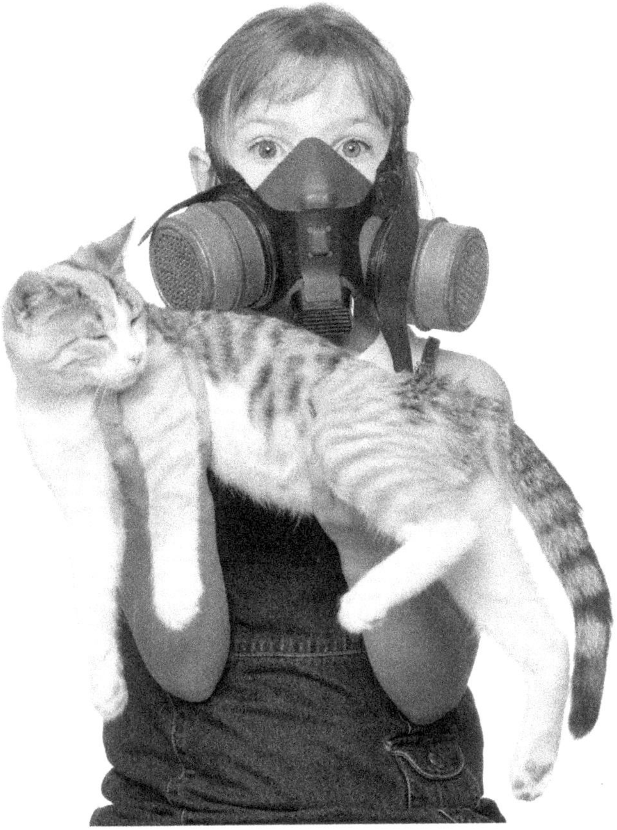

Part 4
Special Considerations

Chapter 25
Ebola Disease in Children

Children can be exposed to Ebola virus if they have contact with the blood or secretions of an animal or person with symptomatic Ebola disease. The risk for children in the United States of being infected with Ebola disease is very low. They have a much greater risk of being infected with influenza than Ebola disease.

Most of what we know about Ebola disease comes from studies related to adults. Statistical information on Ebola disease in children has not been collected. Symptoms of Ebola disease like fever, nausea, vomiting, and diarrhea are common symptoms of illnesses in children year round. Pediatric health care providers must be vigilant in asking about travel to Ebola infected countries or contact with individuals who have Ebola disease. Symptom assessment and prompt laboratory testing is critical for a child who has had potential exposure or traveled in a country where the disease is widespread.

Limited data suggest that children with Ebola disease are more prone toward respiratory and gastrointestinal symptoms. They have higher fevers. They have less central nervous system involvement and experience lower rates of hemorrhage. Children younger than five may be at increased risk of infection and death from Ebola disease. There are no studies or statistical data available on the risk of Ebola disease in infants or in breastfed babies.

Children have lower fluid reserves in their bodies than adults and are more likely to become severely dehydrated from diarrhea and vomiting. They have less blood volume and small amounts of hemorrhage can be very serious.

Early assessment and rapid intervention are critical for successfully managing the care of children with Ebola disease.

There are no vaccines or treatment regimens for children with Ebola disease. Any child diagnosed with Ebola disease should be in the hospital. He should receive supportive care which includes oral or intravenous fluids, oxygen, blood products, and antibiotics when co-infections are suspected. Personal protective equipment (PPE) must be worn by all care providers and strict infection control measures will used. Parents or family members that provide physical and emotional care to the child must also wear PPE. Isolation and quarantine protocols are used to prevent transmission to people who are not sick.

Recommendations to prevent transmission of the Ebola virus:

- Wash your hands often with soap and water for 20 seconds.
- Avoid touching your eyes, nose, and mouth with unwashed hands.
- Avoid close contact like kissing, hugging, and sharing cups and utensils with people who are sick.
- Disinfect surfaces such as countertops, doorknobs, sinks, and toilets to prevent spread of illnesses.
- Sanitize equipment and toys often.
- Separate contaminated clothing and bedding from regular laundry. These items should be washed separately using regular "hot" or "cold" washing cycles and normal drying cycles.
- Most commercial sanitizers, disinfectants, and bleaches will kill Ebola virus. Agents that are effective and instructions for their use can be found on the CDC website.
- Gloves should be used whenever contact with blood or body fluids is anticipated such as changing diapers or soiled linens. The gloves must be removed carefully and disposed of properly to avoid contact with body fluids. Hand washing using correct technique should always follow glove removal.
- Any child who is sick should not attend school or church. He should remain home until he is well again.

- Any child who was exposed to the blood or body fluids of someone with Ebola disease needs to be monitored for 21 days after the last exposure to look for symptoms of Ebola disease.
- A child who is West African is no more likely than any other child to be infected with Ebola disease. This disease infects individuals with exposure to Ebola- not any specific racial or ethnic group.

Discussing Ebola disease with children: Remember- if your child seems anxious and concerned- he really is. You need to find out what he knows and how he feels so you can initiate a conversation with him and reassure him

- Be cautious about discussing Ebola disease where children may overhear.
- Use reliable sources to check the facts on Ebola disease such as the CDC, the WHO, your pediatrician, or the public health department.
- Limit your child's exposure to news programs and social media.
- Ask your child what he has heard about Ebola disease. Listen for underlying fears and concerns and don't downplay or minimize them.
- When children have questions- listen carefully to what they are saying and answer their questions in a clear and direct manner.
- Be honest with your child. Give him the facts.
- Make sure your explanations are age-appropriate.
- Speak in a calm manner and give reassure children that they are safe.
- Assure him that our health care system is among the best in the world for taking care of sick people.
- Help him understand that the risk in the United States is much less than the risk in Western Africa.
- Reassure him that very few people have caught Ebola disease from someone else in the United States.
- Encourage him that doctors and scientists who know a lot about the disease are working hard to find ways to prevent and cure Ebola disease.

- Maintain your child's normal routine. Make sure he gets enough rest and exercise. Provide him with nutritious foods.
- Encourage your child to express himself creatively by drawing pictures and journaling.
- Encourage prayer and quiet time to reflect on his thoughts and feelings.
- Give your child practical advice to help him stay healthy. Reinforce hand washing, hygiene, and healthy living.
- Help him to feel empowered and understand there are things he can do to make a difference.

These are some age-specific behaviors that may signal that a child is feeling fearful and anxious. Children who show these behaviors may need more parental reassurance and support. Any change in behavior that lasts more than 2-3 weeks or seems to be getting worse may benefit from interventions with medical care providers or counselors.

Age 0-2- Infants and toddlers cannot understand what is wrong but they can detect anxiety and fear in their parents and siblings and can express anxiety and uncertainty in non-verbal ways and by regressive behaviors. Thumb-sucking and bedwetting after they have been successfully potty trained are common behaviors when toddlers feel anxious. They may cry for no reason and cling to people they know. They may seem fearful of sickness, strangers, darkness, and monsters. They may not want to play with toys or use high chairs, playpens, or swings. They may refuse to sleep in their beds and cry uncontrollably when left alone.

Cuddle your infant or toddler often. Get down on his eye level and speak in a calm, gentle voice. Use words he understands to soothe and comfort him. Tell him that you love him and will take care of him. Help him feel safe. Keep his normal routine for eating and bedtime.

Age 3-5- Preschool children may want to stay in a place where they feel safe. They will depend on parents and siblings to reassure them and make them feel better. Some may have questions and want to talk about the outbreak. Others may express their understanding through their play or tell exaggerated stories about it. Eating and sleeping habits may change. They may have aches and pains that can't be explained.

Stay close and available but let your child set the tone for how you respond to the Ebola crisis with him. Cuddle him and show your love freely and in ways that are comfortable for him. Be calm and gentle and use words he understands. Answer his specific questions but don't go off on rabbit trails or introduce information he is not ready to hear. Make him feel safe and loved. Encourage him to come to you with questions or when he feels worried or scared.

Age 6-10- Young school age children may want more attention from parents and caregivers. They may show attention-seeking behaviors and have difficulty focusing. Some refuse to do chores or obey instructions. They may fear going to school and stop doing their homework assignments. Their school performance may lag. They may avoid friends and refuse to play. They may act younger than their age and want to be fed or dressed by a parent. They may feel guilty that they are in a place that is safer than the children in Western Africa. They may become aggressive for no reason and express anger and rage.

Comfort your child and ask what worries him and what will make him feel better. Help him to think through and express his feelings. Spend time with him and offer gentle words of encouragement and love. Hug him and help him feel safe and accepted. Keep his routine consistent. Encourage him to spend time with friends and do things he enjoys.

Age 11- 19- Adolescents are going through a lot of physical, emotional, and hormonal changes. They may have a stronger emotional response than a younger child. They may deny how they really feel about Ebola disease to their families and themselves. They may respond "I'm okay" or be silent when they really are anxious and upset. They may have trouble verbalizing their feelings or dealing with anxiety because they think they are adults and should be able to handle it well. They may experience physical symptoms as a result of anxiety. Some may start arguments or be rebellious at home or school. They may resist structure or authority. They may engage in risky behaviors like smoking, drinking, or drug use.

Let your adolescent child set the tone for how to discuss Ebola disease and how to support him. His age and maturity may mean that he will not bring his concerns to you easily. He may brush you off or act like he knows all about it. His response to you may be negative or belittling especially if he is a teen. Honor your child's wishes and support him in the way he needs.

Use this crisis as a way to open the lines of communication with your teen and connect in a way that sustains you as he continues to mature and gain independence.

<u>Warning Signs-</u> Parents should watch for behaviors in their child that may indicate the need for evaluation and intervention by a health care provider or counsellor. When behaviors are uncommon for a child and persist for an unusually long time they indicate that he is not coping adequately. Some behaviors that could be red-flags would include aggressiveness, hyperactivity, speech difficulties, withdrawal, violent behavior, and blatant disobedience.

Your goal is to help your child feel connected, cared about, and loved. You need to be his calm port in the storm during the Ebola crisis. Pay attention to your child and be a good observer. Listen to what he says verbally but also what his behavior says. Encourage questions and honest dialogue. Be caring, committed, and compassionate. Allow him to express himself in his unique way. Do not give up on him even when his behavior is difficult to understand or hurtful. Use this stressful time as a time of growth in your relationship with him.

Chapter 26
Ebola Disease in Pets

Animals that live in Western Africa have the greatest risk of being infected with Ebola disease. Certain animals are known to transmit Ebola virus but not all species that are capable of acting as reservoirs have been identified. Fruit bats, antelope, possums, monkeys, apes, and gorillas have tested positive for Ebola disease in Guinea, Liberia, Sierra Leone, and Mali. Animals living in the African bush have the highest risk of transmitting Ebola virus. There is no evidence that mosquitos, spiders, or insects transmit Ebola virus.

Transmission of Ebola virus requires contact with the secretions of an animal or person infected with Ebola disease who is symptomatic. Animals that are infected will not act in a normal way and will seem very sick. **Ebola virus is not spread by casual contact with a healthy animal.**

Household pets in the United States and in areas of the world that do not have widespread Ebola disease are at very low risk. A pet must have exposure to the secretions of an animal or person with Ebola disease to get infected. The greatest risk of Ebola infection in a household pet would be from an owner who has symptomatic Ebola disease.

This is the joint response of the CDC, The US Department of Agriculture, and the American Veterinary Medical Association about the risk of Ebola disease in pets in the United States:

- There have been no reports of dogs or cats becoming sick with Ebola disease- even in Western Africa where the disease is widespread.
- There is limited evidence that dogs can get Ebola virus but no evidence that they develop Ebola disease.

- There are no reports of Ebola disease being spread from a pet to a person.
- No domestic animals in the United Sates have been diagnosed with Ebola disease.
- The risk of Ebola disease affecting large numbers of American citizens is very low and the risk to domestic animals and pets is even lower.
- No one knows if Ebola can be transmitted on the body, hair, fur, or paws of an animal who has been exposed to the blood or secretions of a person with Ebola disease. Animals should not have contact with potentially infectious blood and secretions when anyone in the household has viral symptoms. They should not lick or roll in potentially infectious secretions.
- When animals live in the household of someone with Ebola disease- the animal should be evaluated by public health officials in collaboration with a veterinarian to determine the level of exposure and look at the general health of the animal. These experts will determine how the pet should be handled on a case-by-case basis according to local and state statutes and guidelines.
- Routine testing for Ebola disease in pets is not available. There is no reason to test any animal who has not been exposed to a person with Ebola disease.
- CDC regulations require that any animals imported into the United States are healthy. They must be vaccinated for rabies before they enter the United States. Each state and U.S. Territory has its own rules for pet ownership and importation and they can be different from the CDC guidelines. Airlines may also have additional requirements for pets to travel on airlines.
- Monkeys can be infected with Ebola disease. They should not be allowed to have contact with anyone who has Ebola disease. Healthy monkeys already living in the United States who have not had exposure to someone with Ebola disease cannot spread Ebola virus.
- African monkeys, rodents, and bats cannot be imported as pets under any circumstances.

- Bats in the United States are not known to carry Ebola disease but they can carry and transmit rabies and other diseases. Never attempt to touch a bat whether it is alive or dead.

The take home message from animal care authorities is that your pet has very little risk of Ebola exposure and that no animals in the United States have been diagnosed with Ebola disease. Take reasonable precautions for your pet's safety and health while continuing to enjoy his companionship and love.

Chapter 27
Ebola Disaster Survival Kits

There is very little risk of Ebola disease in the United States but widespread Ebola disease in the United States would be a real medical disaster. Some degree of foresight and preparation is reasonable. Certain supplies are more unique to Ebola survival than to any other disaster you will encounter. Ebola pandemic kits are already hard to find on Amazon. Sales of protective clothing, goggles, and face masks have gone up over 140,000%. Anyone who waits until the last moment to prepare for an Ebola disaster will be too late. If widespread Ebola disaster were to happen in the United States-protective equipment would be out-of-stock and unavailable. I will begin with a list of emergency supplies that are specific to a medical disaster like Ebola- but then I will focus on guidelines for family disaster plans meant for any type of disaster.

An Ebola disaster kit should include:

- Vitamins including B, C, D-3, E, and B-25
- Superfoods like cranberries, sea weed, and algae
- Supplements like zinc, selenium
- Anti-viral herbs like Echinacea, ginger root, and black elderberry
- Potassium Iodide capsules
- Gauze bandages, Band-Aids, and butterfly closures
- Non-prescription drugs, pain relievers, stomach remedies, and anti-diarrheal
- Thermometers
- Stethoscope, blood pressure cuff, diabetic testing kit and supplies
- Fluid with electrolytes
- Full-body Tyvek suits
- PAPR respirators
- N- 95 or N-100 respirators
- Nitrile exam gloves

- Full face shield
- Safety goggles
- Boot or shoe covers
- Plastic disposable aprons
- Bars of soap
- Alcohol-based hand sanitizers
- EPA-approved disinfecting wipes
- Household bleach
- Disinfectant sprays
- Alcohol
- Hydrogen Peroxide
- Antiseptic solutions and antibiotic creams
- Betadine
- Benadryl
- Baby wipes
- Diapers for infants and toddlers
- Feminine hygiene products
- Regular disposable gloves
- Heavy-duty reusable gloves
- Small trash cans with lids
- Heavy duty garbage bags
- Plastic sheeting
- Ziploc bags of different sizes
- Portable toilet with disposal liners
- Toilet paper
- Paper towels
- Duct tape

- Entertainment for the family like cards, board games, coloring books, pencils and pens, and paper, video games, videos, and books

Recommendations for Family Disaster Plans:

Every family should have a basic first-aid kit and some emergency supplies available. Disasters can happen at any time and trying to stock up and provide for your family's needs during a disaster is a disaster in itself. Survival necessities will disappear from the shelves rapidly and people will fight over them and resort to pushing, shoving, and hurting others. Prepare ahead and check your supplies every month to make sure they are in good condition. Review their expiration dates and replace supplies as needed.

Consider the specific needs of every family member. Make sure you have adequate amounts of medications, food, and clothing for each individual family member and for any pets.

Every family should have an emergency preparedness plan. Each family member should help prepare the disaster plan and it should be reviewed by the whole family every month. Each family member should know their role in a disaster. Everyone should know what to bring and where to meet. All supplies and documents should be kept in a designated place. Nothing should be moved or taken from the kit. Responding to a disaster should be as simple as pick up the kit and walk out the door. Planning and preparation are the keys to calm and efficient execution of the plan during a disaster.

These are the basics that should be included in a disaster survival kit:

- Water- one gallon per person per day
- Food- three day supply of non-perishable food for each person
- Battery operated or hand-crank radio with extra batteries
- NOAA Weather Radio with tone alert and extra batteries
- Battery operated alarm clock
- Flashlight with extra batteries
- First-aid kit and first aid book
- Emergency whistles for each family member
- Basic tools like wrenches, pliers, hammers

- Manual can opener
- Fire extinguisher
- Matches in a water-proof container
- Mess kits, paper plates and cups, plastic utensils, paper towels, toilet paper
- Local and state maps
- Signal flares
- Compass
- Cell phone with charger, inverter, or solar charger
- Important family documents- identification, birth certificates, passports, bank account records, and copies of insurance policies in a waterproof, portable container
- Cash or travelers checks
- Change

Clothing and Bedding: Everyone must remain warm and could be exposed to rain, snow, sleet, or hazardous weather conditions. Several complete changes of warm clothing are essential to layer based on weather conditions and change as needed. Other supplies to include:

- Jacket or coat
- Rain gear
- Long pants
- Long sleeved shirts
- Hat and gloves
- Sturdy shoes
- Weatherproof boots
- Sleeping bag or warm blanket for each family member
- Tent

Prescriptions and medications for each family member:

- Adequate amounts of prescription medications for a week
- Insulin, syringes, alcohol wipes, testing supplies for diabetics

- Contraception and condoms
- Prescription eyeglasses and sunglasses
- Dentures and a denture cup
- Pet supplies including medications, food, and treats
- Mild pain relievers like Tylenol or Motrin
- Anti-diarrheal medications
- Anti-nausea medications
- Antibiotics
- Vitamins
- Cough syrups and cold medicines
- Eye drops and allergy medications
- Insect repellants
- Poison ivy treatment
- Snake bite kit
- Epinephrine Pen
- CPR mask

Toiletries and supplies for personal grooming for each family member:

- Infant formula and diapers
- Feminine hygiene supplies
- Toothbrushes, toothpaste, and dental floss
- Deodorant
- Shampoo and hair care products
- Soap or body wash
- Body lotions and moisturizers
- Suntan lotion
- Towels and washcloths
- Garbage bags and plastic ties
- Moist towelettes, q-tips, and cotton balls
- Band-Aids of various sizes

- Antiseptic ointment
- Petroleum jelly
- Bengay or pain relieving rubs
- Eye ointments and chap stick

These are the golden rules for disaster planning:

- Have the whole family participate and assign tasks
- Prepare everything you need before you need it
- Store your supplies in a designated area known to every family member
- The whole family should review the plan and check supplies once a month
- Go out and enjoy your life while praying that you never need to use your survival kit

Conclusion

There is an Ebola pandemic in Western Africa. Five times more people have died in the 2014 crisis than the total of all deaths attributed to Ebola in history. Ebola is primarily a disease linked to poverty, isolation, and ignorance.

The African people have endured war and genocide for many years. They are suspicious of the motives of governments, police agencies, and even health care organizations. They are ignorant about how Ebola virus is transmitted and what to do to protect their family from disease. Many run from health authorities and hide family members who are sick so they are not taken to hospitals.

The success of our relief efforts in Western Africa will dictate whether Ebola disease spreads throughout the world. If we can break the chain of transmission in West Africa- the pandemic will run its course and stop in Africa. If we are not successful in containing Ebola virus in West Africa- impoverished third world countries with primitive living conditions, poor sanitation, and inadequate medical care will also be at risk of infection with Ebola virus and Ebola will continue to spread.

These are fundamental truths about the Ebola crisis of 2014:

- Ebola disease is wide-spread and under-reported in West African villages.
- Families are hiding their Ebola infected loved ones to keep them in the village with their family.
- Ebola disease is pandemic in Western Africa and it has spread into large population centers in Guinea, Liberia, Sierra Leone, and Mali.
- Porous country borders and easily accessible inter-continental flights will make it very hard to isolate and contain Ebola disease in Western Africa.
- The risk of Ebola disease spreading to other countries and nations of the world increases daily as cases of Ebola disease increase.
- It takes only one lapse in preventive procedures to allow an Ebola infected traveler to leave Western Africa and bring the disease to other countries of the world.

This is the bottom line when we talk about containing Ebola disease in Africa and preventing a global outbreak. It will take the coordinated efforts and co-operation of all nations in the world to succeed in stopping Ebola disease. The global community must lay aside politics and prejudice and unite as one. Diplomacy and effective communication are critical components of any humanitarian effort. Every nation of the world is at risk of Ebola- so every nation of the world must be involved in relief efforts. Nations who are blessed with financial resources and excellent medical care systems should be the first in line to commit humanitarian aid and resources in Western Africa.

The risk of widespread Ebola disease in the United States or in other countries with strong public health organizations and technologically advanced medical care is very low but not zero. The greatest risk will be in health care workers who take care of patients with Ebola disease and humanitarian aid workers who go on medical missions to Western Africa. These are the people who have the greatest risk of direct contact with the blood and body fluids of patients with Ebola disease. These are the true heroes in the Ebola crisis. Gratefully thank them for their service and care for them in their need.

Here are some final thoughts and conclusions about Ebola disease:

- There are no antiviral medications that treat Ebola disease.
- Antibiotics are ineffective against Ebola disease unless there are co-existing infections.
- There is no cure for Ebola disease.
- There are no FDA-approved vaccines to prevent Ebola disease although several are under investigation.
- You cannot get Ebola from a handshake or a hug.
- Ebola virus only spreads if someone with Ebola disease has symptoms.
- Ebola's incubation period is 2-21 days but most who are infected will start to have symptoms by 8-10 days after their exposure.
- Traveling on commercial airlines is safe.
- Ebola is not an airborne disease.
- You will not get Ebola disease from food or water.
- If you are sick- influenza is much more likely than Ebola.

- Washing your hands with soap and water or alcohol-based hand sanitizers is the most effective way to prevent Ebola disease.
- Household bleach and most other disinfectants kill Ebola virus.
- You cannot get Ebola virus from mosquitos, spiders, snakes, or insects.
- Your dog and cat do not transmit Ebola virus and will not get sick with Ebola disease.
- People who are from West African countries or cultures are no more likely to get Ebola disease than you are.
- Body fluids such as blood, feces, vomit, urine, saliva, sweat, semen, vaginal secretions and breast milk can transmit Ebola virus in someone with symptomatic Ebola disease.
- Men who recover from Ebola disease can transmit Ebola virus in semen for up to 7 weeks after they recover. Male survivors should not have sexual relations for three months after recovery.
- The bodies of animals and people who die from Ebola disease are very infectious and do transmit Ebola virus.
- Personal protective equipment (PPE) acts as a barrier that protects the wearer from Ebola virus exposure.
- The CDC website is a comprehensive collection of information, facts, guidelines, and recommendations that is continually updated and current.
- The CDC's Emergency Operations Center is active and available for emergency consultation at (770)-488-7100.

This is a summary of what we know about Ebola. The crisis is very different for citizens of Western Africa than for citizens living anywhere else in the world. Stopping Ebola will require the cooperation and involvement of every country and nation. Africa is like a lit match with smoldering embers in the grass. We must extinguish the flame, put out the fire, and save the world.

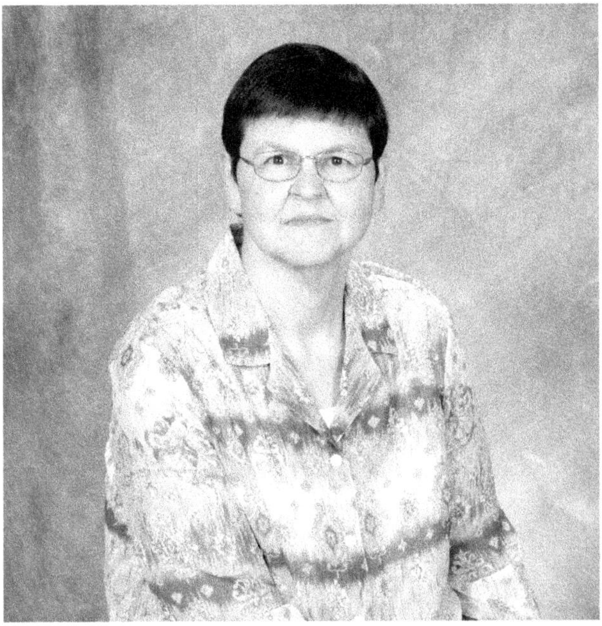

About the Author

Georgia Begnaud has had master's level training in nursing and is a Certified Nurse Midwife. She loves birth and babies and has delivered over 3450 beautiful healthy babies in her 30 year career. Georgia describes herself as being absurdly fascinated with disease and disaster. She studied epidemiology and infectious diseases extensively during her master's program at Columbia University and brings that education and expertise to this book about Ebola disease. It summarizes our current knowledge of Ebola in a straight forward and easy to understand manner. It serves as a framework to help you understand the Ebola pandemic that is unfolding in Western Africa and decide on a response for your family based on the risks of Ebola disease where you live. Georgia can be reached by email for questions and comments at GeorgiaBegnaud@gmail.com.

www.ingramcontent.com/pod-product-compliance
Lightning Source LLC
Chambersburg PA
CBHW051714170526
45167CB00002B/660
9781505553321